DAILY VAGUS NERVE EXERCISES

Revitalize Your Well-being: Unlock Vitality and Inner Balance
with Daily Vagus Nerve Exercises

Michael Stratch

Table of Contents

INTRODUCTION 7

Disclaimer 7

Understanding the Vagus Nerve and Its Role in Well-being......................8

The Science Behind Vagus Nerve Stimulation 9

CHAPTER 1: **YOUR WELL-BEING JOURNEY BEGINS** 10

This book is for you if… 10

The Modern Balancing Act: Work, Family, and Stress............................11

CHAPTER 2: **THE VAGUS NERVE UNVEILED** 16

Anatomy and Functions: Navigating the Vagus Nerve's Complex Pathway 16

In the Head 16

In the Neck...16

In the Thorax 17

In the Abdomen 17

How the Vagus Nerve Regulates Stress and Anxiety 17

CHAPTER 3: **DAILY VAGUS NERVE EXERCISES: A COMPREHENSIVE GUIDE** 20

Quick and Simple: Time-efficient Exercises for Your Busy Schedule 20

Breathing Exercises 20

Yoga...24

Anti-Inflammatory Yoga Poses 28

Kundalini Yoga 30

Bedtime Yoga Routine..31

Chanting..32

Ear Exercises 33

The Salamander Exercises 35

Abdominal Massage 37

Foot Massage 38

Visceral Massage 39

Neck Massage 40

Rib Cage Massage 40

Loving-Kindness Meditation 41

Sleep Meditation 42

Gargling 43

ADAPTING TO LIFE'S DEMANDS: FLEXIBILITY IN APPLICATION 44

SEAMLESS INTEGRATION: INCORPORATING EXERCISES INTO DAILY ACTIVITIES 45

CHAPTER 4: BEYOND THE PHYSICAL: MINDFULNESS AND SELF-CARE **50**

BEYOND THE BODY: INTRODUCING MINDFULNESS AND SELF-CARE TECHNIQUES 50

Mindfulness 50

Self-Care Techniques to Complement Vagus Nerve Activation 51

GUIDED MINDFULNESS EXERCISES: ANCHORING YOUR PRESENT MOMENT 51

Mindful Breath Awareness 52

A 5-4-3-2-1 Exercise 53

Body Scan Meditation 53

Mindful Walking 54

Gratitude Journaling 55

Self-Compassion Break 56

Mindful Eating 57

Body-Focused Meditation 58

CHAPTER 5: THE JOURNEY TOWARDS LASTING WELL-BEING **60**

CUMULATIVE BENEFITS: HOW CONSISTENCY LEADS TO REDUCED STRESS AND ENHANCED MOOD 60

SETTING GOALS AND TRACKING PROGRESS: YOUR PATH TO WELL-BEING 61

CHAPTER 6: TAILORING YOUR APPROACH **66**

DIVERSE TECHNIQUES FOR DIVERSE PREFERENCES: BREATHING, MOVEMENT, AND GROUNDING 66

COMMUNICATION AND CONNECTION: SHARING YOUR SELF-CARE NEEDS 67

CHAPTER 7: EMBRACING A HOLISTIC LIFESTYLE **69**

THE CONNECTION: VAGUS NERVE HEALTH AND HOLISTIC WELL-BEING 69

NURTURING YOUR BODY, MIND, AND SPIRIT 70

CHAPTER 8: **ENHANCING YOUR KNOWLEDGE** **72**

SAFEGUARDING YOUR JOURNEY: ESSENTIAL SAFETY PRECAUTIONS 72

STAYING GROUNDED: NAVIGATING THROUGH MISCONCEPTIONS 73

CHAPTER 9: **THE POWER OF PERSONAL STORIES** **76**

REAL-LIFE ANECDOTES: HOW VAGUS NERVE EXERCISES TRANSFORMED LIVES................76

INSPIRING CHANGE: SHARING YOUR WELLNESS JOURNEY 77

CHAPTER 10: **EVOLVING THROUGH FEEDBACK AND GROWTH** **79**

HONORING YOUR WELL-BEING: ADDRESSING FEEDBACK AND CONCERNS......................79

YOUR EMPOWERING JOURNEY: EMBRACING A LIFELONG COMMITMENT 81

CONCLUSION: EMPOWERING YOUR INNER BALANCE **83**

Introduction

Disclaimer

The information given here are just for basic information and not meant as medical advice. It's really important to highlight how crucial it is to talk to a qualified healthcare expert before making any big changes to your health habits. Every individual's health condition is unique, and what might be suitable for one person might not be suitable for another.

Although we try our best to give correct and current information, remember that what we share isn't a replacement for expert medical advice, diagnosis, or treatment. If you're unsure about a medical issue, it's vital to consult a qualified doctor. Don't ignore professional medical advice or wait to get it just because of what you've seen or read here.

Health-related decisions should be made in consultation with a healthcare professional who has access to your complete medical history and understands your specific health needs. They can provide personalized recommendations that take into consideration your individual circumstances, medical history, current medications, allergies, and any potential interactions.

Remember that medical information and practices are constantly evolving, and what may be considered accurate today could change in the future. So, it's crucial to stay well-informed by referring to reliable sources and trusting the knowledge of qualified healthcare professionals when making informed choices about your well-being.

Understanding the Vagus Nerve and Its Role in Well-being

The vagus nerve functions as a vital communication pathway within the body, facilitating the exchange of information between the brain and internal organs. At times of rest and relaxation, it's in charge of modulating the reactions of the body. This important nerve begins its journey in the brain and travels down through the neck and body in a number of different routes. It carries out functions such as relaying sensory information from the ear's skin, controlling the muscles involved in swallowing and speaking, and influencing the immune system. Known as the tenth cranial nerve (CN X), the vagus nerve is the longest mixed cranial nerve. Despite its singular reference, it consists of a pair of nerves emerging from both sides of the medulla oblongata in the brain stem. Its name, "vagus," translates to 'wanderer,' accurately reflecting its extensive connections with the cortex, brainstem, hypothalamus, and the body. Approximately 80% of its pathways are afferent (sensory), while the remaining 20% are efferent (motor).

This nerve forms the sensory network that informs the brain about the status of various organs, particularly the digestive tract (including the stomach and intestines), as well as the heart, lungs, spleen, liver, kidneys, and numerous other nerves that impact activities such as speech, eye contact, facial expressions, and even the capability to interpret others' voices. Comprising countless fibers, its operations occur at a level below conscious awareness, yet it plays a crucial role in maintaining overall well-being. As an integral component of the parasympathetic nervous system, it counteracts the "fight-or-flight" stress response by calming organs after exposure to danger.

The vagus nerve's distribution is extensive, serving several functions:

- **Sensory:** It also controls the innermost parts of the laryngopharynx and the larynx. The skin of the auditory canal on the outside is also innervated by it. In spite of this, it offers the organs of the abdomen and heart the capacity for sensory experience.
- **Special Sensory:** It is responsible for providing the epiglottis and the base of the tongue with a feeling of taste.
- **Motor:** The vast bulk of the muscles that make up the pharynx, soft palate, and larynx receive motor innervation from this nerve.
- **Parasympathetic:** In addition to controlling the rhythm of the heart, it provides innervation to the smooth muscles of the gastrointestinal system, the trachea, and the bronchi. Its cardiac branches cause the heart beat to slow down, while its bronchial branches cause the bronchi to narrow, and its esophageal branches control the involuntary

muscles in the esophagus, stomach, gallbladder, pancreas, and small intestine. These limbs encourage the digestive process known as peristalsis as well as the release of digestive chemicals.

The Science Behind Vagus Nerve Stimulation

The vagus nerve is an essential part of the human nervous system. It travels a circuitous route from the brain all the way down past the face, the thorax, and finally into the abdomen. This nerve originates in the medulla oblongata of the brain, which is located within the brainstem. It then travels laterally before leaving the cranium via the jugular foramen. It then continues downhill into the carotid sheath, until it lies posteriorly and to the side of the inner and ordinary carotid arteries, whilst resting medially to the inner jugular vein. This is because its continuing path takes it lower inside the carotid sheath. When it reaches the base of the neck, the vagus nerve splits into two branches that go in separate directions through the thorax, one branch going to the right side of the chest and the other to the left.

The journey of the right vagus nerve into the thorax is characterized by its passage across the initial segment of the subclavian artery, posterior to the innominate artery. Subsequently, it navigates behind the primary right bronchus and the esophagus, ultimately converging with the left vagus nerve to create the esophageal plexus. On the other hand, the left vagus nerve travels into the thorax via going through the left common carotid artery and the left subclavian artery. This is how it enters the chest cavity. As it continues down its path, it winds up passing behind the primary left bronchus and entering the esophagus, where it joins forces with its counterpart.

A noteworthy point of intersection occurs within this intricate pathway, where the accessory nerve (also known as cranial nerve XI) converges with the vagus nerve. This union transpires just beyond the inferior ganglion, further contributing to the network of neural connections and signaling.

The vagus nerve takes an intricate route through the body, originating from the brainstem's medulla oblongata, exiting the skull through the jugular foramen, and proceeding downwards within the carotid sheath. Upon entering the thorax, it follows distinct trajectories for the right and left sides. The right vagus nerve journeys behind arteries and bronchi to form an esophageal plexus with its counterpart, while the left vagus nerve takes an alternative route behind different vessels and bronchi to ultimately join the esophagus. This neural journey is also marked by the accessory nerve's integration into the vagus nerve's course. This complex pathway highlights the intricate connectivity of the nervous system and its role in regulating numerous bodily functions, comprising those associated to the heart, lungs, and digestive system.

Chapter 1

Your Well-being Journey Begins

This book is for you if...

This book is for you if...

- You're a health enthusiast who's already dedicated to your well-being journey and wants to dive deeper into the science and techniques of vagus nerve exercises.

- You're a stressed professional caught in the fast-paced modern world, seeking effective stress-reduction strategies provided in the book.

- You're a mind-body wellness seeker who believes in the deep connection between your physical and mental well-being. The book's holistic approach aligns with your quest for a harmonious understanding of your body and mind.

- You're a holistic practitioner in alternative therapies, looking to enhance your knowledge with a scientifically grounded foundation. This book can expand your toolkit and provide more comprehensive support for your clients.

- You're actively searching for ways to achieve emotional balance. If you're dealing with anxiety, mood swings, or emotional imbalances, the book offers practical solutions for your well-being.

- You're a wellness coach, educator, or instructor within the wellness industry. The book's evidence-based insights can seamlessly enrich your teachings and improve the guidance you provide to your clients.

Value Proposition for the Target Audience

This book offers a multifaceted value proposition that resonates with the diverse target audience:

- **Scientific Understanding:** For health enthusiasts and professionals alike, the book provides a solid scientific foundation. It explains the anatomical and physiological aspects of the vagus nerve, ensuring readers understand the mechanisms behind the exercises.
- **Practical Techniques:** The book doesn't just offer theoretical knowledge; it's a practical guide. It introduces readers to a variety of exercises – from deep breathing and meditation to gentle yoga poses – that can be easily integrated into daily routines.
- **Stress Reduction:** Stress is a common factor in modern lives, affecting both mental and physical health. The book equips stressed professionals and individuals seeking emotional balance with effective tools to manage stress and promote relaxation.
- **Holistic Approach:** The book aligns with the holistic perspective shared by mind-body wellness seekers. It acknowledges the interconnectedness of various bodily systems and offers exercises that address both physical and emotional well-being.
- **Personal Empowerment:** "Daily Vagus Nerve Exercises" empowers readers to take control of their health. By providing a clear roadmap and step-by-step instructions, the book encourages readers to become active participants in their well-being journey.
- **Customization:** The book recognizes that everyone's well-being journey is unique. It offers a range of exercises, allowing readers to choose those that resonate most with them, fostering a sense of customization and personalization.
- **Integration with Existing Practices:** For holistic practitioners and wellness coaches, the book complements existing knowledge and practices. It introduces a scientifically grounded approach to enhance the services they provide to their clients.

The Modern Balancing Act: Work, Family, and Stress

In the contemporary landscape, the demands of work, family, and personal well-being often intertwine, creating a delicate dance that individuals must master to maintain a fulfilling and harmonious life. The interplay of these three fundamental aspects – work, family, and personal needs – constitutes a multifaceted challenge that shapes the way we navigate our daily lives. This section explores the intricate dynamics that arise from the interplay of these domains and examines the strategies that can help individuals navigate this complex balancing act successfully.

Work

In the modern world, work is a cornerstone of identity, financial stability, and personal growth. However, the demands of the professional realm can permeate other areas of life, impacting personal time, relationships, and overall well-being.

1. **Time Commitment:** Work often commands a significant portion of our waking hours. The traditional 9-to-5 workday can stretch longer due to extended hours, commuting, and the increasing expectation of being reachable outside office hours.

2. **Career Advancement:** Ambitions for career growth and success can drive individuals to invest extra time and effort into their work. This pursuit, while fulfilling, can potentially upset the equilibrium between work and personal life.

3. **Work-Related Stress:** Pressures such as deadlines, performance expectations, and work-related conflicts can trigger stress, which can have ripple effects across personal and family life.

4. **Technological Impact:** The advent of technology has transformed work dynamics, allowing constant connectivity. While fostering flexibility, it can blur the lines between work and personal time.

Family

Family, whether nuclear or extended, forms the foundation of support, love, and social connections. However, maintaining these relationships alongside other obligations presents a unique set of challenges.

1. **Caregiving Roles:** Parenting, spousal duties, and caring for elderly family members demand time and emotional energy. These responsibilities can sometimes conflict with professional obligations.

2. **Quality Time:** Finding quality time to nurture relationships within the family is essential. However, the pressures of work and external commitments can limit the availability of such moments.

3. **Support Network:** Family often serves as a vital support network, helping individuals cope with challenges. Balancing these relationships can be particularly demanding during times of stress.

4. **Flexibility:** The need to accommodate family needs, unexpected events, and emergencies requires a degree of flexibility that can sometimes clash with rigid work schedules.

Personal Needs

Amid the demands of work and family, the pursuit of personal well-being can often take a backseat. Neglecting one's own needs can lead to burnout, stress, and a decline in overall physical and mental health.

1. **Self-Care:** Prioritizing self-care activities, such as exercise, relaxation, hobbies, and creative outlets, can contribute to emotional well-being and resilience.

2. **Time for Reflection:** Personal growth requires time for introspection and self-discovery. Balancing this with external demands is essential for maintaining a sense of identity and purpose.

3. **Mental and Emotional Health:** Nurturing mental and emotional health is crucial. Neglecting self-care can lead to stress-related conditions, impacting work, family relationships, and overall quality of life.

4. **Leisure and Hobbies:** Engaging in leisure activities and hobbies provides a healthy outlet for stress and fosters a sense of fulfillment beyond work and family roles.

Challenges of the Balancing Act

The modern balancing act presents a complex set of challenges that individuals must navigate:

1. **Time Constraints:** With the demands of work and family, finding time for self-care and leisure activities becomes a challenge. The 24-hour day feels insufficient to fulfill all responsibilities.

2. **Emotional Toll:** Balancing multiple roles can result in emotional exhaustion. Meeting the needs and expectations of both the workplace and family can leave individuals drained.

3. **Guilt and Expectations:** Many individuals grapple with guilt, feeling torn between their work commitments and family obligations. Societal and personal expectations can exacerbate this sense of guilt.

4. **Boundary Blurring:** The advent of technology blurs the boundaries between work and personal life. Constant connectivity makes it difficult to fully disconnect from work during personal time.

5. **Neglected Well-Being:** The pursuit of balance often leads to the neglect of personal well-being. Lack of self-care can lead to stress, burnout, and a decline in overall health.

Strategies for Navigating the Balancing Act

While achieving a perfect balance may be elusive, adopting strategic approaches can help individuals navigate the challenges:

1. **Prioritize:** Identify your top priorities in work, family, and personal well-being. Focus on these priorities to allocate time and energy more effectively.

2. **Set Boundaries:** Create distinct boundaries between your business time and your leisure time. Maintaining a healthy balance requires that you communicate these limits to your coworkers, family members, as well as yourself.

3. **Delegate:** It is important to not be scared of delegating chores at work and to include family members in the obligations of maintaining the household. Sharing the load lightens the burden and allows for more balanced time management.

4. **Time Management:** Embrace effective time management techniques, such as the Pomodoro Technique or time blocking, to assign precise time slots for work, family, and personal activities.

5. **Practice Self-Care:** Prioritize self-care by engaging in activities that rejuvenate your mind and body. Regular exercise, meditation, and hobbies can contribute to your overall well-being.

6. **Disconnect Mindfully:** Set designated times for checking work emails and messages. Outside those times, disconnect from work devices to create mental space for personal and family time.

7. **Embrace Flexibility:** Recognize that achieving balance may require flexibility. Some days, work demands might take precedence, while other days, family needs may require more attention.

The ability to navigate the modern balancing act goes beyond mere time management. It involves cultivating resilience and adaptability. Life is dynamic, and circumstances change. Developing the ability to adjust and adapt to new situations is essential for maintaining balance and well-being.

Chapter 2:

The Vagus Nerve Unveiled

Anatomy and Functions: Navigating the Vagus Nerve's Complex Pathway

The cranial nerve also known as the vagus nerve possesses the most extensive pathway among all cranial nerves, stretching from the head to the abdomen. Its designation originates from the Latin term 'vagary,' signifying wandering. It is occasionally denoted as the "wandering nerve."

In the Head
The medulla of the brainstem is where the vagus nerve starts its journey. It exits the skull by passing through the jugular foramen, alongside the glossopharyngeal and accessory nerves (CN IX and XI correspondingly). Inside the skull, the auricular branch emerges, responsible for providing feeling to the back portion of the outer ear canal and the external ear.

In the Neck
In the region of the neck, the vagus nerve enters the carotid sheath and proceeds downward alongside the internal jugular vein and the common carotid artery. As they reach the lower neck, the right and left vagus nerves take distinct paths:

- The right vagus nerve courses in front of the subclavian artery and behind the sternoclavicular joint before entering the thoracic region.
- The left vagus nerve travels down between the left common carotid and left subclavian arteries, positioned behind the sternoclavicular joint, and proceeds into the thoracic region.

Numerous branches originate in the neck:

- Pharyngeal branches: A significant portion of the pharyngeal and soft palate muscles receive their motor input from these branches.
- Superior laryngeal nerve: This nerve gives off branches that go both within and outside the body. Although the internal branch gives sensory impulses to the laryngopharynx and the upper region of the larynx, the outside branch is responsible for providing innervation to the cricothyroid muscle in the larynx.

- Recurrent laryngeal nerve (on the right side only): After making a loop below the right subclavian artery, this nerve continues its journey upward towards the larynx. It is responsible for providing innervation to the majority of the larynx's intrinsic muscles.

In the Thorax
Within the thoracic region, the right vagus nerve gives rise to the posterior vagal trunk, while the left vagus nerve gives rise to the anterior vagal trunk. These vagal trunks emit branches that add to the creation of the oesophageal plexus, responsible for innervating the smooth muscle within the esophagus. Additionally, two other branches emerge in the thoracic area:

1. The left recurrent laryngeal nerve, which curves beneath the arch of the aorta and ascends to provide innervation for the majority of intrinsic muscles within the larynx.

2. Cardiac branches that are responsible for regulating heart rate and offering visceral sensation to the heart.

Entering the abdominal region through an opening in the diaphragm known as the oesophageal hiatus, the vagal trunks continue their course.

In the Abdomen
Within the abdominal region, the vagal trunks conclude their course by splitting into smaller branches that deliver innervation to the esophagus, stomach, and both the small and large intestines (extending as far as the splenic flexure).

How the Vagus Nerve Regulates Stress and Anxiety

The vagus nerve, a complex cranial nerve with far-reaching connections, plays a pivotal role in regulating stress and anxiety within the human body. Emerging research highlights its profound influence on the autonomic nervous system, emotional regulation, and overall well-being.

Central to its role in regulating stress and anxiety is the autonomic nervous system, a division of the peripheral nervous system that manages automatic bodily functions. The vagus nerve plays a key role in this system, harmonizing a nuanced equilibrium between the sympathetic and parasympathetic branches. The sympathetic branch fuels the well-known "fight or flight" response, triggering stress and anxiety in response to perceived threats. In contrast, the parasympathetic branch activates the "rest and digest" response, promoting relaxation and calmness. The vagus nerve primarily engages with the parasympathetic system, acting as a counterbalance to stress and anxiety-inducing signals.

Activation of the vagus nerve sets in motion a cascade of physiological changes that counteract stress. One of its primary effects is the reduction of heart rate and blood pressure. By sending signals to the heart's sinoatrial node, the nerve slows down the heart rate, promoting a state of relaxation. Simultaneously, the vagus nerve influences blood vessel dilation, leading to decreased blood pressure. These combined effects contribute to an overall sense of calmness and well-being.

Furthermore, the vagus nerve is intrinsically linked to the brain's emotional centers, such as the amygdala and the prefrontal cortex. The amygdala, responsible for processing emotions and fear responses, receives inhibitory signals from the vagus nerve. This dampens the amygdala's reactivity, reducing the intensity of emotional responses to stressors. Meanwhile, the prefrontal cortex, which governs executive functions and emotional regulation, communicates bidirectionally with the vagus nerve. This interaction helps modulate emotional responses and enables a person to better manage anxiety-provoking situations.

Neurotransmitters also play a vital role in the vagus nerve's stress-regulating effects. Acetylcholine, a neurotransmitter released during vagal activation, has anxiolytic properties, contributing to relaxation and stress reduction. Another neurotransmitter, gamma-aminobutyric acid (GABA), promotes feelings of calmness and tranquility. The vagus nerve's influence on these neurotransmitters adds another layer to its stress and anxiety regulatory mechanisms.

Various techniques and practices have been shown to stimulate the vagus nerve, harnessing its stress-reducing potential. Deep breathing exercises, for instance, enhance vagal activity by increasing the variance between consecutive heartbeats, a phenomenon known as heart rate variability. This heightened variability indicates a balanced autonomic nervous system and a reduced stress response. Mindfulness meditation and yoga also promote vagal stimulation through slow, controlled breathing and heightened body awareness. Physical activity, particularly aerobic exercises, boosts vagal tone, leading to increased parasympathetic activity and reduced stress.

Research into biofeedback and vagus nerve stimulation devices is expanding the realm of possibilities for stress and anxiety management. Biofeedback systems provide real-time information about physiological processes, enabling individuals to consciously influence their autonomic responses. Vagus nerve stimulation devices, which deliver controlled electrical impulses to the nerve, are being explored as potential treatments for anxiety disorders and depression. These innovations hold promise for enhancing our understanding of the vagus nerve's role and its therapeutic applications.

The vagus nerve's intricate web of connections and multifaceted effects culminate in its remarkable ability to regulate stress and anxiety. By promoting parasympathetic activity, interacting with emotional centers in the brain, and influencing neurotransmitter release, the vagus nerve serves as a crucial ally in maintaining emotional equilibrium. The adoption of techniques that stimulate the vagus nerve, along with the exploration of innovative technologies, opens doors to effective stress and anxiety management. As science continues to unveil the complexities of this cranial nerve, its potential to enhance our mental and emotional well-being becomes increasingly evident.

Chapter 3:

Daily Vagus Nerve Exercises: A Comprehensive Guide

Quick and Simple: Time-efficient Exercises for Your Busy Schedule

In this part, we shall discuss several workouts for the vagus nerve and the potential benefits that these exercises may have for an average person in everyday life. In order to activate the vagus nerve and lead a life that is less fraught with tension and anxiety, try performing these easy exercises.

Breathing Exercises

In recent years, notable studies have observed that longer exhalations improve heart rate variability and help the vagus nerve recover so that we are not stuck in a perpetual state of fight-flight-freeze. Heart rate unevenness is the healthy fluctuation in the intervals between heartbeats. All living animals have this.

The breathing cycle has an inhalation and an exhalation phase.

On inhaling, the SNS (sympathetic nervous system) causes a brief heart rate acceleration.

On exhaling, the vagus nerve secretes a substance called Ach that helps send signals from one nerve cell to the next, causing the heartbeat to slow down and consequently activating the PSNS (parasympathetic nervous system)and enabling the rest-and-digest system into action.

Slower breathing, with an added focus on those longer exhalations, can stimulate the vagus nerve and help achieve a strong HRV, according to a review of studies.

Your heart rate variability is a part of the fitness of your vagus nerve, its vagal tone, and the way it responds. A higher HRV is a sign of solid vagus nerve health, which means lower stress, better cognition, and an overall healthy state. Therefore, strengthening your heart rate variability is an excellent way to improve your vagal tone, combat undue stress, and help an overactive nervous system driven by a fight, flight or freeze response.

Breathing techniques to calm and focus the mind are as ancient as civilizations.

These techniques resurface from diverse cultures in the modern day through practices like Yoga and Tai Chi. These practices regularly embrace slow, meditative breathing patterns. They concentrate on moderating how we breathe by gently shifting the breathing to longer exhalations (compared to inhalations), enabling practitioners to identify their natural breathing consciously.

Breathing this way moves awareness to focus on the act of respiration as beginning with the abdomen instead of the upper chest and head. In other words, when you breathe with awareness, you ensure your in-breaths are happening from the stomach, not the nose or chest.

The vagus nerve loves when you breathe well. Breathing well is a simple yet powerful way to tell your body and your vagus nerve that you are okay right now.

It's an effective way to bring more oxygen into your body, help your nerve wake up, and notice that there is no real threat so that it can move from the fight-flight-freeze mode of operation to the rest-and-digest mode.

Breathing correctly literally tells your vagus nerve, "It's okay. We're okay." There's a phrase for this. It's called "respiratory biofeedback." This is your body's built-in method of biofeedback. Breathing enhances the balance of physical, mental, and emotional health, which helps with managing stress and performance. Breathing well is a love letter to your vagus nerve.

Valsalva Maneuver

- Take a deep breath in.
- Now close your mouth, pinch your nose, and gently breathe out.
- Hold this for a moment, and then release your nose to let out your breath.

This technique will create a gentle pressure in the chest cavity, which, in turn, stimulates the vagus nerves connected to the lungs and airways.

Diaphragmatic Breathing

The diaphragm is a bell-shaped muscle located directly beneath the lungs.

When you inhale, the muscle flattens out, acting as a kind of pump to allow the lungs to expand. When you breathe from the diaphragm, you breathe deeply to fill the chest.

You'll notice your stomach expands outward, and contracts when you exhale.

There are two basic ways to breathe from the diaphragm.

The first is to *simply breathe*!

- Sit in a quiet place with your back straight.
- Sit either in a cross-legged position, or with the feet planted firmly on the floor.
- Take a deep breath, making a conscious effort to fill the chest with air.
- Hold it for a moment, and then breathe out. Do this for at least two minutes.

The other way is to *sing*!

- In order for your lungs to get enough air to sing, you must breathe from the diaphragm. So when you start to sing, you automatically breathe from the diaphragm.
- Otherwise, you wouldn't have enough air to push through your vocal cords and no sound would come out.
- Put on a song you like and sing along.

If you do this every day, you're giving your diaphragm a good workout and you're giving your vagus nerve both psychological and physical stimulation.

Audible Breathing

Normally your breath is silent. When your exhale is audible, however, it means that the glottis is partially closed. The glottis is located at the back of your tongue. The vagus nerve is connected to the glottis, and stimulating this part of the tongue stimulates the vagus nerve.

- For audible breathing exercises, find a quiet place to sit with your back straight.
- Sit in a cross-legged position or sit with your feet planted firmly on the floor.
- Take a deep breath and hold it for a moment.
- When you exhale, sigh or hiss out your breath.
- Think of the sound you made as a child to breathe on a cold window in order to fog it up. Breathe in this way for at least two minutes.

7-11 Diaphragmatic Breathing Exercise

- Locate a calm spot to sit, and make sure your back is completely straight.
- Sit with your legs crossed or your feet planted firmly on the floor.
- Inhale through your nose, filling the chest cavity with air, and count to seven.
- Hold your breath for one second, then exhale audibly through the mouth, making a sigh or a hissing sound.

- Exhale for a count of 11.
- This is one cycle. Repeat this for six-12 cycles a day.

Obstructed Diaphragmatic Breathing Exercise

- Locate a calm spot to sit, and make sure your back is completely straight.
- Sit with your legs crossed or your feet planted firmly on the floor.
- Inhale through your nose, filling the chest cavity with air, until you can't take in even one more drop of air.
- Then purse your lips and exhale forcefully, almost as if you are blowing all of the air out of your lungs.

Do this until you can't exhale any more. This is one cycle. Repeat this for 6-12 cycles a day.

Yoga

Yoga is a systematic practice that is related to the mind, body, and spirit. It originated from India. This 5,000-year-old practice has gained momentum across the world, and it is slowly becoming one of the preferred ways to exercise because it doesn't only strengthen the physical body but also eases stress. It also has less impact on joints and muscles, which means it appeals to a wide range of people regardless of age.

Yoga practice involves manipulating your body into various postures, paired with meditation and breathing exercises, thus placing us into the rest-and-digest mode and moving us away from the flight-and-fight mode. There are many benefits to practicing yoga:

- It increases blood flow.
- It supports your spine.
- It drains your lymph.
- It increases immunity.
- It lowers blood pressure.
- It positively impacts mood.
- It helps you get better sleep.

Below are three yoga poses to try at home to boost your vagus nerve:

Savasana

Traditionally speaking, this pose is done at the end of a yoga practice. However, if you struggle with sleeplessness, headache, or stress, then this pose is suggested to help ease the symptoms.

- Simply lie down on a flat surface with your arms alongside you, palms facing upwards.
- Inhale and exhale at your own pace.
- Hold this pose for a count of 20 breaths.

Legs Up The Wall

This pose boosts blood flow through the body, strengthens the immune system, and manages stress.

- Simply lie flat on your back.
- Raise your legs parallel to the wall so that your hips are touching the wall.
- You may keep your knees slightly bent, whatever is most comfortable for you.
- Keep your body relaxed, and stay in this pose for however long you feel is necessary.

Bridge Pose

This pose is important for opening up your chest and supports the immune system in fighting infections.

- Lie on the floor with your knees bent over your ankles.
- With your arms alongside you, palms facing downwards, gently lift your pelvis off the floor.
- Bring your chin to your chest and hold this pose for a count of five breaths.

Sun Salutation

The Sun Salutation, also known as "Surya Namaskar," is a dynamic and invigorating yoga sequence that serves as a foundational practice in many yoga traditions. This sequence is a harmonious combination of postures, breath, and movement, and it is often used to warm up the body and prepare it for a deeper yoga practice. The Sun Salutation is not just a physical exercise; it also holds spiritual significance, symbolizing the gratitude and connection to the sun, which is considered a source of energy and vitality.

- Come to a standing position with your two big toes connected with a slight space between your heels.
- Join your hands in front of your chest.
- Firmly ground your feet to the mat or floor. Inhale and exhale normally.
- Relax your upper back and neck as you inhale and reach your arms up toward the sky. Hold the position for a few seconds, exhale as you bring your arms back to your side.
- Continue the exercise by inhaling as you raise your hands, holding the position, and exhaling as you bring your hands back to your sides.

Relaxation Asana

The Relaxation Asana is a seated yoga pose focused on relieving tension in the neck muscles and promoting a sense of relaxation.

- Sit in a crossed legged position. Make yourself comfortable.
- Put your hands over your eyes and carefully move your head in a clockwise circular motion.
- While you do this try not to strain your neck. Observe how the muscles in your whole neck stretch out completely.
- Once you have completed rotating the neck in a clockwise direction, start rotating them in a counterclockwise direction.

- Complete three sets of three rotations clockwise and three sets of three rotations counterclockwise.
- You can alternate between clockwise rotation and counterclockwise rotations as well.

Mountain Pose (Tadasana)

Mountain Pose, known as Tadasana, is a foundational yoga posture that cultivates a sense of grounding, alignment, and mindful presence.

- Prepare yourself by coming to a standing position with your feet together. Make sure that your feet are firmly planted on the floor. Loosen your toes by lifting them off the ground, spreading them out like a fan and then dropping them back down on the ground.
- Feel the ground beneath the soles of your feet. This sensation allows you ground your feet firmly to the floor or surface you are standing on.
- You have to now engage your thigh muscles. Lift your knee caps. If you are doing this right, you will feel as though your knees and and calf muscles are tight. If possible, try to do this without hardening your lower belly.
- Stand up straight. You need to have a straight posture.
- Broaden your shoulder span. When executed accurately, you should sense a sense of alignment in your shoulders. Here's a useful trick: if you push your shoulders directly backward, you might experience a slight unease. To enhance the comfort of this motion, begin by raising your shoulders toward your ears and then smoothly rotate them outward and toward the back.
- As you do this, ensure you don't thrust your lower front ribs forward. Instead, elevate the upper part of your sternum and let your arms dangle naturally at your sides.
- Keeping your neck long, with the chin parallel to the floor. Look straight ahead, as though you are focusing in the distance.
- You might find that your jaw muscles have tightened at this point. Relax them. Soften your gaze. You are performing yoga, not getting ready for an MMA match.

Plank

The Plank pose is a foundational yoga posture that focuses on building core strength and stability.

- Lie down face-down on the floor with your arms on either side of your chest. It should look like you are about to perform some push-ups.
- Shift your position so that you are not resting on your forearms, which are now bent at a 90 degree angle at the elbows.
- Now position your elbows directly beneath your shoulders.

- The rest of your body should look like it is in a straight line, from the crown of your head all the way to the heels.

Upward Dog

Upward Dog is a yoga pose that combines strength and flexibility, often used as a transition or component in various yoga sequences.

- Lay down on the ground with your stomach facing up. First, extend your legs behind you, and then put the balls of your feet on the ground. You should squat down with your elbows bent and your palms placed on the ground next to your waist, like you're getting ready to do a push-up.
- Breathe in and push your hands into the floor.
- After that, extend your arms to their full length and, at the identical time, elevate your torso and your legs a couple of centimeters off the ground. At this point you can bend your toes such that the base of your toes are touching the floor.
- Now lift your head up in such a way that it looks as though you are facing forward. Don't try to bend your back too much. Some people can look straight ahead while others can bend even further. You don't have to try anything that makes you uncomfortable. The most important thing to remember is that you have to get the pose right.

Downward Dog

Downward Dog, also known as "Adho Mukha Svanasana" in Sanskrit, is a fundamental yoga pose that is commonly practiced in various yoga styles.

- Lie down on the ground on your hands and knees. Put your knees so that they are squarely under your hips, and move your hands so that they are a little in front of your shoulders.
- Spread your palms, your hands as parallel to each other as possible. Bend your toes that the base of the toes are touching the floor.
- Breathe out and raise your knees off the ground. Start by keeping your knees a little bent and your heels lifted. It will almost look like you are about you launch yourself somewhere! But don't launch yourself anywhere.
- We are going to focus on your tailbone. It is the part that is the bottom of the spine. Lengthen your tailbone and lift your buttocks towards the ceiling. It should seem like you are trying to imitate the letter 'A.'
- Bring your knees into a straight line, but be careful never to lock them. Straighten your hands as well but don't lock your elbows.

Anti-Inflammatory Yoga Poses

Yoga stimulates the vagus nerve through a number of channels. From movements to breathing techniques, it has been one of the most effective ways to strengthen the nerve and trigger it to heal from various health problems. These yoga poses specifically help with management and reduction of symptoms caused by chronic conditions.

Supine Twist

The supine twist pose can help clear away negative energy and pain while also massaging the internal organs. This pose can help increase blood flow to the vital organs, which can reduce inflammation. To perform this pose:

1. Begin in a laying down position on your back.

2. Bring the knees in towards your chest as you inhale and exhale deeply.

3. Slowly twist at the hips so the knees drop to the right side of your body.

4. Bring your arms out to your side so that your body forms a T.

5. Turn your head in the left and hold the pose for five breaths.

6. Bring the knees back up to your chest and perform this on the other side.

Half Lord of the Fishes Pose

This yoga pose utilizes a deeper twist movement, which can help initiate the detoxification of the digestive system. This is a cleansing pose that can help reduce inflammation. To perform this pose:

1. Begin in a seated position on the floor with the legs stretched out in front of you.

2. Bring the right foot up and position it so it sits outside of the left quad.

3. Bring the right foot up and just outside of the right hip. Both hips should remain on the floor.

4. Take the left elbow and rest it on the outside of the right knee while the right hand should be planted gently behind you to provide stability and support.

5. Draw the crown of the head up towards the sky, allowing the spine the lengthen.

6. Hold this pose for five breaths. Then reach the arms up above your head can you stretch the legs back out in front of you. Repeat the steps on the opposite side.

Performing the child's pose can help you reduce anxiety, stress, and fatigue. It is a simple yoga move that uses a slight inversion move that helps stimulate the digestive tract. To perform this pose:

1. Begin with your hands and knees on the floor, in a tabletop-like position. The wrist should be placed just under the shoulders and the knees just under the hips. Knees should be about hip-width apart. The big toes should be touching.

2. Keep the big toes touching as you bring the hips down and back toward the heels of your feet. Your torso should be pressed forward with the abdomen resting between the knees. Stretch the arms out in front of the head with the palms pressed to the ground.

3. Inhale and exhale deeply five times.

Kundalini Yoga

Kundalini yoga is the ideal blend of three different types of yoga: Shakti (the embodiment of strength and vitality), Raja (meditation and the art of mental and physical control), and Bhakti (chanting and devotion). Simply put, the balance of these three provides perfect harmony mentally, physically, and spiritually.

The beauty of this type of yoga is that it leaves you feeling uplifted. It also enables you to embrace yourself and the world around you as it is. For the vagus nerve, this practice is like winning the lottery. In Sanskrit, Kundal means "circular," and in this practice, your spine is depicted as a snake. All energy is focused and based at the bottom of your spine.

When practicing Kundalini yoga, the idea is to stir the snake and have it metaphorically move its way through the six chakras (centers of energy located at specific places in the body) and then through the top of your head (the seventh chakra). Chakras are said to be able to distribute energy throughout the body from their locations. The practice of Kundalini is to tap into these centers and improve overall health.

Below are three Kundalini yoga poses to try at home:

Fire Breath

This pose holds detoxifying elements that spread warmth throughout the body using a simple breathing technique.

- On a flat surface, take a seat, crossing your legs comfortably.
- Inhale deeply through your nose, extending your abdomen outward as you do so.
- As you exhale, pull your stomach inward and toward your spine, breathing out once again through your nose.
- Remember to keep your spine straight and your arms resting comfortably atop you knees.

Archer

Boost your determination and encourage confidence with this pose.

- Stand in an upright position.
- With your left foot, firmly step back.
- Keep your right knee slightly bent.
- Raise your right arm parallel to your body as if holding the front end of a bow.
- Hold your left arm in line with your right as if you are pulling an imaginary bow string.
- Both hands are kept in soft fists.

- The pose should resemble that of an archer at the ready as indicated.

Ego Exit

On an even surface, sit with your legs crossed comfortably and spine straightened. Raise each arm into the air at a 160-degree angle and point only your thumbs upward into the air. Your fingers should be gently folded at the knuckles in a semi-fist pose. Begin with the fire breath technique. This pose is useful because it opens up the heart and cleans the lungs out.

Bedtime Yoga Routine

Yoga is far less strenuous than running around the block or pumping weights in the gym; hence, it can help you relax and unwind. Moreover, it can dissolve pent-up stress that occurred throughout your day and can ease the mind. It is highly recommended that you either practice a routine or hold a few poses before bedtime.

This sequence will guide you through various poses that aid in digestion, calm the mind, and relax the body. To boost sleep, hold each position for one minute.

1. ***Butterfly***

Sit comfortably, spine upright. Place the soles of your feet together and clasp them together with your hands, knees bent. Continuously press your knees toward the mat. Remember to breathe and to keep your back straight.

2. ***Head to knees***

As you remain seated in the butterfly position, bring your legs out in front of you. As you exhale, try to clasp your feet with your hands or rest them mid-leg, whatever is most comfortable for you. Gently bring your head down to rest on your knees or as close as you can.

3. ***Twist***

Sit upright with your legs still straightened in front of you. With your right hand placed on your left knee and left hand placed semi-behind, you gently pull the right side of your body to the left. Repeat this from left to right, and remember to breathe. Hold each twist for five breaths.

4. ***Legs up the wall***

Take up this position by lying against the wall, raising your legs parallel to the wall for support (a 90-degree angle). Try to stay in this position for over five minutes.

5. *A simple forward bend*

Take a seat on the floor with your legs crossed. Stretch your hands and arms out in front of you and over your knees, finally resting them on the ground ahead of you. Bring your head down to the floor as far as you can.

6. *Corpse pose*

Recline in an appropriate position on your mat or bed, with your arms and legs stretched out in front of you. You are going to want to close your eyes and concentrate on the breathe in and breathe out. With every breath that you take, focus on a specific area of the body. With every exhale, imagine tension and stress leaving this part of the body.

7. **Continue like this until sleep finds you.**

Chanting
The muscles in your larynx and vocal cords are linked to the vagus nerve. Chanting is a good way to activate the vagus nerve. Using chanting as a mechanism to stimulate your vagus nerve also has a calming effect on the body by helping slow down your heart rate.

To activate your vagus nerve using chanting, the following steps can be used:

1. Sit in a comfortable position in a quiet and well-aerated room.

2. Close your eyes.

3. Have your head, neck, and spine in alignment, but your body should be relaxed not tense.

4. Stretch your spine, and as you do so, tilt your chin towards your chest so that your neck is elongated.

5. The elongating of the neck will serve to stretch the vagus nerve.

6. Relax your throat so that the vibrations of your chant are distributed around the neck.

7. Inhale deeply focusing on feeling the air enter your body.

8. Then as you exhale, make the 'Oom' sound without.

9. As you chant, do not use force or tense your diaphragm.

10. Repeat the inhale followed by the exhale with the 'Oom' sound ensuring that your throat stays relaxed.

Humming and singing are also easy ways to activate your vagus nerve. Ever noticed how good you feel singing in the shower? Well, the secret to the feel-good effect is the stimulation of the vagus nerve. Singing is versatile, and you can do it while stuck in traffic by singing along to your favorite music. Singing is an instant mood lifter and an effective way to activate your vagus nerve and put your body in a relaxed state.

Ear Exercises

Although you may not think your ear can be stiff, they can get slightly tight if you have not reached a vagal tone. The vagus nerve branches to the ear, and these are called the auricular branches. To see whether you are in a vagal tone, try pulling your ears away from the skull. Usually, one ear may feel a little tighter than the other. Notice how soft or firm your ears feel when pulling. Take note of whether you can move it up and down and how that feels like. Once you tested for vagal tone through your ear, you can go ahead and do this exercise. You can check back with this technique after doing the exercise to see if your ears are a little less tight afterward.

1. You need to start by accessing the hollow part of the ear located above the ridge of your ear close to your ear canal. Slide your finger into the hollow above the ridge and gently apply a circular motion. You are not required to press hard at this area but rather think of moving the skin around in circles. Very little pressure is needed for this exercise. Whilst doing this exercise, you may experience changes in your breathing; you may sigh or swallow. Once you are done from one side, repeat the same process on the other ear. You may start to experience a feeling of calmness, but this is not obligatory. You may experience such physiological symptoms when massaging one ear but experience no changes when massaging the other side. There is no strict time limit for this exercise. Feel free to spend as much time as you wish.

The vagus nerve can be accessed at the ear but from a different area. Here is how:

2. An alternative way to stimulate the vagus nerve is at the back of your ear canal. Once you find the back of your ear canal, with your index finger, you must press towards the back of your head whilst making little circles to massage the area. The same principle here applies, so there is no need to press but rather move the skin in the area in circular motions. This movement gives sensory information to your nervous system. Applying extra force is not

productive in this instance. Once you are done with one side, go ahead and repeat the same technique to the other ear. Just like the previous exercise, you may notice that one side is easier to massage than the other, and that is where you would confirm that you are not in a vagal tone. It is important to notice these little details whilst massaging. For this technique, there is also no stipulated time limit, so you can keep at it for as long as you wish.

3. Another way to massage your ears to stimulate your vagus nerve is using this technique. Take your ear and give it a gentle stretch. This focuses on stretching the entire ear around without using excessive force. This is very beneficial if you have temporomandibular (TMJ) issues. This area refers to the sliding connector of your jawbone to the skull. This is found on each side of the jaw. TMJ issues can be caused by injury to teeth, bruxism, poor posture, stress, or arthritis. If you suffer from stress headaches, this might be especially helpful. Pull your ear gently down and away from your skull during the exercise. This sends sensory information to your nervous system that creates a calming response. Once you are done with one side, repeat the same on the other ear. You may feel like it is painful on one side but painless on the other. If this is the case, do not practice this exercise on the painful side because this would make this exercise counterproductive.

4. Take the skin behind your ear and your hairline and gently slide it up towards the top of your head. Focus on stretching the skin behind your ear upwards. This should be done to the skin only, so no force is required. Stretch the skin for a while whilst you hold for a few seconds. This is sending sensory information to your brain. This helps your brain to realize that the muscles in that area can move, in turn releasing that area. Once you are done pulling the skin up, take the same area and pull it down towards your neck and away from the top of your head. Hold the stretch in both directions. Do the same technique but pull towards the back of your head. Repeat the same technique to the other side. As with the previous exercises for the ears, there is no stipulated time for which you must keep at this exercise. You may notice that one movement is easier than the others on one side. This is very common, and it is suggested that you repeat the exercise towards the directions where your skin moves more easily because it is more productive and effective.

After executing these techniques, feel free to check for tightness in your ears, as suggested above. These exercises may provide a release of tightness around the neck and the jaw. Your eyes may feel softer whilst breathing is easier through the sinuses. You can use this technique for instant stress and anxiety relief.

The Salamander Exercises

The following "Salamander Exercises" gradually increase flexibility in the thoracic spine, freeing up movement between the individual ribs and the sternum in the joints. It will increase your breathing capacity, help reduce a forward head posture by getting your head back into better alignment and reduce scoliosis (abnormal spine curvature).

Eighty percent of the vagus nerve fibers are afferent (sensory) fibers, meaning they bring back information from the body to the brain. Only 20 percent are efferent (motor) fibers that carry the brain's instructions to the body. Some of the afferent fibers from CN IX and CN X sections monitor the amount of oxygen, and carbon dioxide found in the blood. By improving our breathing pattern with these exercises, we're telling the brain (via afferent nerves) that we're safe and our visceral organs are working correctly. It, in turn, encourages development in the ventral vagus.

But what comes first? Is a reduced breathing pattern product of a dysfunctional ventral vagus, or is input from a less than adequate breathing pattern caused by a lack of ventral vagus function? Suppose there are tensions in the pulmonary diaphragm and the muscles that shift the ribs. In that case, input from the afferent vagal nerves controlling such movements can indicate irregular breathing, avoiding a state of ventral vagal action, just as restoring ventral vagal activity will boost the physiological condition. Either one is beneficial, regardless of which occurred first.

A forward head position reduces breathing space in the upper chest. The Salamander Exercises can create more space for the heart and the lungs in the upper chest. Reducing a forward-head stance will also relieve friction from the nerves entering the spinal cord's heart, lungs, and digestive organs. The Salamander Exercises can alleviate pressure on vertebral arteries by strengthening the cervical vertebrae's positioning and reducing specific back pains between the arms.

You raise your brain to the same level as the rest of your body when doing the Salamander Exercises. This pose is similar to that of a salamander. It does not have a tail, so its head is like an additional vertebra at the tip of the spine. A salamander cannot stretch, extend, twist, or side-bend his head independently about the spine's first vertebra, or lift his head above the spinal vertebra point, as reptiles and mammals can. This exercise is done in line with the spine with the head.

Such exercises put your head in a position that is neither up nor down in your spinal movements. The thoracic (the chest part of the spine) can now bend horizontally, somewhat like a salamander.

In your thoracic vertebrae, you may use side-bending motions to relieve muscle tension between your ribs and the thoracic spine. It makes the lungs move freely and encourages healthy breathing.

There is typically greater flexibility in the neck and lumbar vertebrae in the expansion and flexion of the human spine and less flexibility in the thoracic spine. However, with side-bending, the thoracic spine's strength increases dramatically. The thoracic vertebrae facet joints are opened, making for a freer side-bend of the thoracic spine.

Level 1: The Half-Salamander Exercise

To do the Salamander exercise, sit or stand in a comfortable position in the first part to the right.

- Make your eyes look to the right without turning your head.
- Continue to face forward, turn your head to the right so that your right ear moves closer to your right shoulder without raising your shoulder to meet it
- Hold your head for thirty to sixty seconds in this position.
- Then let your mind get neutral again, and change your eyes to look forward again.
- On the other hand, do the same now: let your eyes look to the left, then tilt your head to the left. After thirty to sixty seconds, return your head to an upright position and your eyes towards a forward target.

The Half-Salamander—A Variation

Follow the exact instructions in this variant of the Half-Salamander exercise, but let your eyes look to the right when turning your head to the left. When you move your head, turning your eyes in the opposite direction increases your range of motion; you should be able to bend your head even further to the side. Hold this for thirty to sixty seconds, then turn back to the other side to do the same thing.

Level 2: The Full Salamander Exercise

The movement on Full Salamander includes side-bending the entire spine rather than just the neck. It uses another body position, too.

- Get down on all fours, protecting your knees and hand palms with your weight. You can rest your hands on the floor, but it's better if you put your hand palms on a desktop, table, chair seat, or sofa pillows. Your eyes should be on the same plane as your neck
- In this exercise, your ears should not be raised above your spine or below that point. Lift your head slightly above what you think is right to find the correct head position. You should be able to feel the head raised slightly. Then, slightly lower your head under what

you think is right. You should know that the head is below what it should be. In between the two positions, go back and forth. Put a little of your head up and take it down a little. Try to find a halfway place where the head doesn't move too far up or down. Even though you might never immediately reach the spot, you will start to zero in on it.

- Once you have found a good head position relative to your back, look right with your eyes, keep them in that position, and turn your head sideways to the right by turning your right ear towards your right shoulder.
- Complete the turn by allowing the curve in your side to extend past your jaw down to your backbone.
- Hold this position for 30 to 60 seconds.
- Put the spine back to the center.
- Repeat all the above steps, but on the left.

Abdominal Massage

Applying a small amount of pressure on the abdomen can help reduce the release of inflammatory cytokines while also calming the nervous system. Through this simple massage technique, you can activate the vagus nerve and increase bowel movement in the digestive tract. This exercise can be performed on yourself and is most effective if it has been a few hours since you last ate. This massage should be performed daily over a four- to six-week timespan as it can help trigger the anti-inflammatory response while also improving digestion, reducing stress, and minimizing the pain that is common with chronic illnesses.

Abdominal massage steps:

1. Lie down on your bed or floor mat.

2. Find your breast bone, or sternum, and place your hands just below this area. Using both your hands, one after the other, begin to massage the area in downward strokes that move towards the abdomen. Continue this downward stroking for two minutes.

3. Then starting towards the side of your abdomen, use your fingers to create small massaging circles. Apply as much pressure that still feels comfortable. Move from the sides of the abdomen inwards while working downwards. Continue this massaging technique until you have covered the whole area of the abdomen.

4. When you have finished, continue to lay on your back. Bring your knees towards the chest and gently rock just the lower half of your body from side to side, resting for 30 seconds on each side, twisting at the hips/abdomen area.

Foot Massage
A foot massage has the ability to bring forth a state of deep relaxation. Furthermore, your feet have the distinct sensation that they're floating on clouds, however they also feel so good that they could possibly tap dance all the way till dawn.

In addition to the amazing physical feelings, getting a massage can also help your vagus nerve, which is an important aspect of your autonomic nervous system. When you massage the feet, you are stimulating important nerves that are associated to the sympathetic nervous system and the parasympathetic nervous system. This causes the heart rate to slow down. A foot massage offers support to the vagus nerve, which, in spite of assisting in the slowing of your pulse rate, also offers support to the vagus nerve. You now possess a potent combination that is directed toward creating about a state of relaxation within you. Let's have a peek at some effective techniques for giving your feet a massage.

When it comes to massage, lotion is a great option to have at your disposal. Prior to you start the massage, rub it into your palms and take a deep breath of the aroma.

1. When you've reached a state of relaxation, tightly grasp one of your feet with both of your hands. Applying light pressure in a circular motion with your thumbs, rub the top of the foot. Just one of your thumbs should be used for the massage.

2. Begin at the very end of every individual toe, and then gradually work your way up toward the ankle. When you reach the ankle, move back towards the toes. Perform this step a total of two or three times. You are more than welcome to repeat what you just said if you so choose.

3. Continue holding your foot. Now you are going to use your middle and ring finger to massage the base of your foot.

4. Begin at the very end of every individual toe, and then gradually work from there up to the heel of the foot.

5. If you are sensitive to being tickled, it is recommended that you apply a massage oil. The ticklish effect is mitigated as a result of the oil, which keeps your fingers from coming into direct touch with your skin.

6. Once you've worked your way up to the heel, you can begin working your way back up to your toes. Perform this step a total of two or three times. You are more than welcome to repeat what you just said if you so choose.

7. Now repeat the previous two steps on the other foot.

We will be shifting our focus to the toes at this point.

1. Grab the foot using one hand, gripping it around the middle.

2. With the other hand, grip your big toe by putting your thumb on top of it and your index finger underneath it.

3. Give the toe a little twist and a gentle pull till your fingers can slide all the way to the end of the toe. As soon as you have reached the very end of the toe, bring your thumb and index finger all the way back to the beginning.

4. Follow the same process with each of the toes.

5. Do the identical steps on your other foot.

Visceral Massage
Massaging the organs below your diaphragm can help stimulate the vagus nerve. You require a core ball and a yoga block for this exercise.

Lay down with your head on the yoga block with the core ball under the side of your abdomen. You may benefit from this exercise more if you expose your skin, so take off your shirt or tuck it up for this exercise. Whilst the core ball is under the side of your abdomen, slowly move on your side and let your abdomen slide over the core ball. Your fatty tissue and visceral organs should be on the core ball whilst your hand is over this area to encourage this. Your hand is now acting as a heavyweight on your abdomen. During this technique, apply the deep breathing technique. You should observe your stomach rising and falling as you breathe. After a while at this exercise, you should start hearing sounds coming from your gut and that represent digestion. It is a clear sign that this exercise is working and your vagus nerve is stimulated. This technique helps to move gas down the sigmoid area of the intestines and out when laying down on the left. When turning to your right, digested food is encouraged to move through the intestines. Allow a few minutes on each side for this exercise.

Neck Massage
Using a core ball against the neck exerts pressure which in turn stimulates your vagus nerve. This exercise can activate the relaxation response.

Place the core ball against the side of your neck, just under your ears. Spin the ball around your neck, and make sure you roll it against soft tissue lining the neck. The movement should be as if you are shaving off a beard but with the core ball instead of a blade. You should be moving from one side below the ear to the other side. As you are crossing your neck with the core ball, you are going to go over your larynx and trachea. These areas are a little more sensitive to pressure than the rest of your neck. When you reach this area, release the pressure slightly. Restore the pressure once you reach the deeper muscle layers at the side of your neck. You are massaging muscles in the neck, usually overused in cases of stress and anxiety. When the ball reaches the lateral muscles of the neck, the pressure applied affects the carotid artery. This artery goes into the carotid sinus that is innervated by the vagus nerve. The pressure applied by the core ball is going to slow down the heart rate and breath pace hence inducing a relaxation response. You should practice this exercise for a couple of minutes while moving from one side to the other several times. Once you remove the core ball, you should feel a warming sensation returning to your neck. After a while, your facial muscles should feel like they are softening. The vagus response initiated by this exercise also impacts the muscles of the face, head, and neck. You may notice that your hearing and your eyesight improves after this exercise.

Rib Cage Massage
For this exercise, you need a yoga block and a small core ball. This is going to help you stimulate the vagus nerve via its connections at the diaphragm and lungs.

1. Place your head on the yoga block and the core ball underneath your ribcage and lay on one side. For the purpose of the exercise, the core ball needs to be between your armpit and the first ribs. Take your other hand and put it on top of the ribcage. This step requires you to have some internal rotation on that shoulder, but if you struggle with this, place a pillow on that side and let your arm hang down instead. This can still provide some sort of pressure to the side, similarly to placing your arm on top of the ribcage. Inhale and hold the breathe whilst contracting your muscles in the ribcage. This can seem like you are trying to cough, but you are not. Exhale and allow your breath to exit your body. Rest until you feel like you need to breathe again. Breath in again as you expand your ribs and hold your breath. During the breathing phase, your ribs should feel like they are expanding to accommodate

the exaggerated breaths you are taking during this exercise. This allows you to feel your heartbeat. This exercise is relaxing for the nervous system, which in turn stimulates the vagus nerve.

2. Another exercise using the same equipment requires you to lay face down with the small core ball placed under your sternum. The yoga block is not required in this exercise. Lay with your face flat on the ground with your arms crossed over and placed under your head. This exercise activates the heart's natural pacemaker, the sinoatrial node. Similar to the previous exercise, breath in and hold your breath whilst pretending to cough. Release the breath and wait until you feel like you need to breathe again to inhale. If you are prone to anxiety, you may want to repeat this exercise for ten to twenty minutes. If you suffer from panic attacks, this is a great way to flip your stress response, settle down, feel calmer, collected, and in order.

Loving-Kindness Meditation
This form of meditation is a favored practice that is used to reach a sense of calm and reduce stress. This form of meditation can open up our tolerance and compassion for others and ourselves. You do not need to be at an expert level to practice this meditation, and it is well suited to those who wish to venture into meditating.

While practicing this meditation, the idea is that you focus on attracting positive and loving thoughts and emotions toward yourself first before wishing the same to those around you and in the far corners of the world. This form of meditation is also said to alleviate depression and anxiety and help those who deal with anger.

This emotion-boosting meditation has its roots firmly planted in Buddhist traditions and practices. While in meditation, you are encouraged to generate feelings of empathy and understanding inward and then outward. Here is how to practice loving-kindness meditation:

- Find a secluded spot for yourself with no interruptions from the outside world. Remember to switch off your phone and all electronic devices if you find yourself indoors. You do not want your meditation to be interrupted, as that would defeat the purpose and end goal.
- Finally, seat yourself comfortably. You can sit or lie down for this exercise. Find a position that will not require you to adjust the pose and interfere with your meditation later on.
- Close your eyes, take deep breaths, and take a moment to center yourself.

- Imagine yourself to experience absolute peace and balance. Understand that you are loved and are perfect the way you are. With every inhale, imagine positive feelings to enter your body. With every exhale, imagine that tension and stress are leaving your body.
- Repeat the following sentences silently to yourself:
- "You can and will be happy."
- "You can and will be safe."
- "You are healthy, loving, and strong."
- "You will receive and give kindness today."
- Soak in these affirmations and feelings of positivity.
- Focus on your breath and the affirmations.
- At your own time, move your focus to wishing peace, love, and joy onto those closest to you, such as family and close friends.
- Once you have focused your best intention upon yourself and loved ones, move your attention to wishing only good health and prosperity for those who also come into contact with you during your day.
- Gradually expand to wishing health, peace, and love unto all those in the world.
- When you feel that you have spent enough time on your meditation, you may open your eyes and gently bring yourself to awareness.
- It is suggested that you revisit the feelings that you had during your meditation throughout your day.

Tip: You can set yourself a gentle alarm to rouse you from your meditation if you only have a few minutes a day to commit to the practice. The above meditation is only a guideline to the practice, and you are welcome to change it to suit your needs.

Sleep Meditation
This meditation, apart from stimulating the vagus nerve, has the added benefit of promoting sleep. By choosing to follow this meditation, you open yourself up to getting rid of unwanted thoughts that might hamper your chances of drifting off to sleep.

Mindfulness teaches us to reflect on the present moment and to view things as they are, no less and no more. When undertaking sleep meditation, there is nothing to force, nor is there any that needs to occur. Just be. There is no end time; rather, the result of this is a blissful night's rest.

1. Begin by lying down in your bed, your arms gently resting beside you or placed onto your stomach, legs slightly apart, which is most comfortable for you.

2. Notice your breath, the rise and fall of your chest, the feeling of fullness in your lungs, and the air passing through your nose and mouth.

3. Let your thoughts wander, but do not heed them. Let them pass with each exhale.

4. Cast thoughts of criticism and judgment aside. Breathe them out with every exhale. In the present moment, there is nothing that needs your attention.

5. Move on to paying attention to your body and your senses. Slowly work your way from the tips of your toes to your feet, legs, all the way up to your head. Concentrate on the way each body part feels and registers while meditating. Release any tensions you might feel in areas such as the shoulders or hips.

6. Pay attention to the feeling of the blanket against your skin or the way it feels under the palms of your hands. Pay attention to the weight of your head as it rests on the pillow.

7. If you find yourself still awake at this time, shift your attention back to your breathing. Inhale and exhale for a few more minutes.

8. After a while, you can begin to count your breaths — *in, one; out, two*. When you reach 10, repeat the cycle.

9. Enjoy a peaceful night's rest!

Gargling

Gargling is an act of bubbling liquid in the mouth by breathing through it with a gurgling sound. It is known as a home remedy for certain conditions, including sore throat, mouth sores, canker sores, allergic reactions, respiratory infections, and other conditions that affect the throat and mouth.

Although no valid research has been carried out into the effect of gargling on the vagus nerve, it is believed by many experts that gargling may help in activating the vagus nerve. This is because gargling contracts the muscles at the back of the throat, thus activating the vagus nerve and stimulating the gastrointestinal tract. Also, the physical reverberation of the vocal cords can activate the vagus nerve, according to D'Elia Assenza. Since gargling causes this reverberation, then it can be employed to stimulate the vagus nerve.

To gargle, pour yourself a cup of water, tilt your head back, and pour some of the water - a quantity that you are comfortable with- into your mouth without drinking it. Try to keep your epiglottis closed during this period to prevent drinking the water. Gargle the water vigorously for anywhere between 20 and 30 seconds before swallowing the water.

Pour some more water from the cup into your mouth and repeat the process for another 20 or 30 seconds. Repeat this cycle until the cup is empty. If you do it right, you might feel yourself begin to tear up. If you do not tear up, we encourage you to keep gargling until you can feel yourself begin to tear up a little bit.

You should gargle about four or five times daily and for long periods to ensure its effectiveness in stimulating your vagus nerve.

Adapting to Life's Demands: Flexibility in Application

Adapting to life's demands requires a holistic approach. Incorporating daily vagus nerve exercises into one's routine is a valuable strategy for promoting resilience and well-being. Here are some tips for successful integration:

1. **Consistency**: Consistency is key. Commit to a specific time each day to practice vagus nerve exercises, whether it's during your morning routine, a lunch break, or before bedtime.

2. **Start Slowly**: If you're new to vagus nerve exercises, start with simple techniques and gradually incorporate more complex ones as you become comfortable.

3. **Mindful Practice**: Engage in exercises with mindful awareness. Focus on the sensations and responses in your body as you perform each exercise.

4. **Variety**: Experiment with a variety of distinct workouts to figure out which ones work most effectively for you. Variety not only keeps your routine interesting but also ensures that you target the vagus nerve from various angles.

5. **Combine Approaches**: Consider combining different exercise approaches for a comprehensive effect. For instance, start your day with deep breathing, incorporate mindfulness during breaks, and end with a calming yoga session.

Seamless Integration: Incorporating Exercises into Daily Activities

Incorporating vagus nerve exercises into your daily routine can help you achieve optimal vagal tone. However, it's important to consider a few key factors when integrating these exercises. The main goal of your routine is consistency, so be sure to blend these practices seamlessly into your comfort zone. Avoid overloading your day with too many activities, as this might lead to incomplete tasks and loss of motivation. Success should be your guide, ensuring that you can accomplish your daily tasks effortlessly.

Begin by introducing a few simple elements into your daily life. This way, the changes will feel minimal, and you'll be stimulating your vagus nerve without disrupting your routine. However, remember that this doesn't mean excluding other activities and methods. As you become more accustomed to specific practices, explore ways to incorporate additional ones. It's important to note that not all exercises need to be performed daily.

Morning Routine:

1. **Breathing Exercises:** Start your day with deep breathing exercises like the **7-11 Diaphragmatic Breathing Exercise** or **Obstructed Diaphragmatic Breathing Exercise**. These can help oxygenate your body, reduce stress, and increase alertness.

2. **Yoga Poses:** Begin your morning with some gentle yoga poses like **Mountain Pose (Tadasana)** and **Child's Pose** to stretch and wake up your body.

3. **Chanting:** If you're inclined, incorporate a few minutes of chanting or mantra repetition to set a positive tone for the day.

4. **Morning Walk:** While walking, perform **Audible Breathing** to focus on your breath and clear your mind.

Throughout the Day:

1. **Foot Massage:** During breaks, give yourself a quick foot massage to relax and rejuvenate.

2. **Abdominal Massage:** Incorporate abdominal massage techniques before or after meals to aid digestion and alleviate discomfort.

3. **Chanting:** Whenever you need a mental break, engage in some soothing chanting to center yourself.

Afternoon or Evening Routine:

1. **Anti-Inflammatory Yoga Poses:** In the afternoon or evening, practice **Supine Twist** and **Half Lord of the Fishes Pose** to release tension from the spine and boost circulation.

2. **Breathing Exercises:** Perform the **Valsalva Maneuver** to enhance your lung capacity and support respiratory health.

3. **Yoga Asanas:** Engage in a sequence of yoga asanas like **Sun Salutation, Plank, Upward Dog**, and **Downward Dog** for a balanced workout.

4. **Kundalini Yoga:** Incorporate **Fire Breath** and **Archer Pose** to invigorate your energy and focus.

Evening Routine:

1. **Loving-Kindness Meditation:** Before bed, practice a short session of loving-kindness meditation to cultivate compassion and relaxation.

2. **Sleep Meditation:** Wind down with a sleep meditation session, incorporating deep breathing and mindfulness to prepare your mind for restful sleep.

3. **Bedtime Yoga Routine:** Follow the **Bedtime Yoga Routine** you've listed, moving through gentle poses like **Butterfly, Legs up the Wall**, and **Corpse Pose** to promote relaxation.

4. **The Salamander Exercises:** Include **The Half-Salamander Exercise** and **Full Salamander Exercise** as part of your evening stretching routine.

5. **Gargling:** Before brushing your teeth at night, incorporate gargling to promote oral health.

Weekly or Intermittent:

1. **Visceral and Neck Massages:** Dedicate a day or two each week for a more thorough **Visceral Massage** and **Neck Massage** session to release tension and promote circulation.

Write here your routine and favourite exercises:

Chapter 4:

Beyond the Physical: Mindfulness and Self-Care

Beyond the Body: Introducing Mindfulness and Self-Care Techniques

Incorporating mindfulness and self-care techniques into your daily routine can be a powerful way to mitigate stress and promote the health of your vagus nerve. In this section, we will discuss a variety of techniques to consider, each designed to cultivate a sense of calm, support your vagus nerve, and enhance your overall quality of life.

Mindfulness
Mindfulness is a process through which you become aware of your body, relaxing deeply and allowing your body to go through its thought processes without interruption or influence. When you go through mindfulness, you are effectively meditating, and doing so can have fantastic results on your mental health. This sort of meditation can directly influence your state of mind, helping to cope with depression and anxiety. It can make you happier and more able to focus and function. It can help people cope with pain. It has also been shown to reduce the biomarkers for inflammation.

Now, compare those effects of mindfulness to those that you have learned about thus far through learning about the vagus nerve—they are incredibly similar. Thanks to how similar they are, what happens if the two are connected together?

The answer is that you get increased results. You are able to remain calm while also getting all of the fantastic benefits of stimulating the vagus nerve in the first place. The best way to do this, then, is to utilize vagus nerve stimulation into your mindfulness routine. If you do not have a mindfulness routine already, the following section will give you one to follow while still utilizing vagus nerve activation.

How it Works

Mindfulness allows for the individual to essentially detach from emotions, pain, or anything else that is actively occurring at that moment that is unpleasant or uncomfortable. This means, then, that the individual can better cope with any discomfort. In coping better, the individual can then manage their ability to relax and cope, effectively ensuring that they are able to regulate their heart rate.

Through breathing techniques during mindfulness, you take control of your physical self. This allows you to take deep breaths and directly impact your vagus nerve and therefore heart rate. Doing so then enables you to better regulate, and that is likely where some of the anti-inflammatory benefits of mindfulness come into play.

Self-Care Techniques to Complement Vagus Nerve Activation

1. **Healthy Nutrition:** Fuel your body with nourishing foods that support your overall health. Eat a diet that is well-balanced that contains a lot of lean proteins, whole grains, fruits, and vegetables, as well as healthy fats. Stay away from foods that include too much sugar, caffeine, or processing.

2. **Physical Activity:** Regular exercise can significantly impact your stress levels and vagus nerve health. Engage in activities you enjoy, whether it's brisk walking, yoga, swimming, or dancing. Aim to complete at least half an hour of moderate physical activity on nearly every day of the week.

3. **Quality Sleep:** Give importance to your sleep by setting up a regular sleep timetable and crafting a soothing bedtime routine. Shape your sleeping space to promote restfulness, and target 7-9 hours of good sleep each night.

4. **Social Connections:** Nurture your relationships with friends and family. Engaging in positive social interactions can boost feelings of connection and reduce stress.

5. **Creative Expression:** Engage in creative activities that bring you joy, whether it's painting, playing a musical instrument, or writing. Creative expression can be a cathartic outlet for stress

Guided Mindfulness Exercises: Anchoring Your Present Moment

Guided mindfulness exercises offer a path to find tranquility in the midst of our fast-paced lives. These exercises encourage us to focus our attention on the present moment, fostering a deep awareness of our thoughts, sensations, and surroundings. By engaging our senses, breath, and self-compassion, these practices provide a powerful means to reduce stress, enhance self-awareness, and cultivate a more balanced and peaceful existence

Mindful Breath Awareness
Mindful breath awareness is a mindfulness practice that involves focusing your attention on your breath in a non-judgmental and present-moment manner.

1. **Find a Quiet Space:** Choose a quiet and calm space where you can sit or lie down without interruptions.

2. **Assume a Comfortable Posture:** Sit or lie down in a relaxed and comfortable position. You can sit on a cushion, chair, or on the floor with your back straight but not stiff. Place your hands on your lap or by your sides.

3. **Close Your Eyes:** Gently close your eyes to help reduce external distractions.

4. **Focus on Your Breath:** Begin to observe your breath as you inhale and exhale naturally. Pay attention to the sensations of your breath as it enters and leaves your body.

5. **Stay Present:** As you focus on your breath, your mind might naturally wander. When you notice your thoughts drifting, gently guide your attention back to your breath without self-criticism. Be patient and compassionate with yourself.

6. **Non-Judgmental Awareness:** Approach your breath with non-judgmental awareness. There's no need to label your breath as "good" or "bad." Simply observe it as it is.

7. **Observe Sensations:** Pay attention to the physical feelings of your breath—observe the lifting and lowering of your chest or belly, the refreshing coolness as you inhale, and the comforting warmth as you exhale.

8. **Anchor:** Your breath serves as an anchor to the present moment. At any time that you become aware that your mind is traveling, return your focus again to the breath that you are taking.

9. **Length of Practice:** You can start with a couple of mins and gradually extend the practice to longer durations as you become more comfortable.

10. **Daily Practice:** Consistency is key. Try to incorporate mindful breath awareness into your daily routine, whether it's in the morning, during breaks, or before bed.

A 5-4-3-2-1 Exercise

This exercise uses your senses to ground you in the present moment. It's called the 5-4-3-2-1 exercise because you'll be focusing on different sensory experiences in your environment. Find a quiet place to sit comfortably, and let's begin:

1. **5 Things You Can See**: Open your eyes and take a moment to identify five things around you that you can see. These could be objects, colors, or patterns. Pay close attention to the details of each item.

2. **4 Things You Can Touch**: Now shift your focus to your sense of touch. Identify four things that you can touch or feel around you. This could be the texture of your clothing, the surface of a table, or the sensation of the air on your skin.

3. **3 Things You Can Hear**: Tune in to your sense of hearing. Identify three sounds you can hear in your environment. These might be distant sounds, ambient noises, or even the sound of your own breath.

4. **2 Things You Can Smell**: Pay attention to your sense of smell. Identify two things you can smell, whether it's the scent of a nearby object, the air around you, or any aromas present.

5. **1 Thing You Can Taste**: Finally, bring your attention to your sense of taste. If you have something to taste nearby, take a moment to savor it. If not, you can focus on the taste of your own mouth or even just the sensation of your breath.

As you move through each step, take your time to fully engage with your senses and the sensations they provide. This exercise helps ground you in the present moment and can be particularly helpful when you find your mind racing or feeling overwhelmed.

Body Scan Meditation

This exercise involves a body scan, which helps you connect with your physical sensations and cultivate awareness of your body. Find a comfortable and quiet space to lie down, and let's get started:

1. **Lie Down**: Find a comfortable place to lie down on your back. You can use a yoga mat, blanket, or anything that provides a soft surface.

2. **Close Your Eyes**: Close your eyes gently. Take a few deep breaths to settle into the present moment.

3. **Focus on Your Breath**: Begin by focusing on your breath. Feel the natural rhythm of your breath as you inhale and exhale. Allow your breath to be your anchor to the present moment.

4. **Start the Body Scan**: Begin to shift your attention to your body. Start at the top of your head and slowly move your focus down through each part of your body. As you do this, notice any sensations, tensions, or areas of relaxation.

5. **Observe Sensations**: As you scan through each body part, observe any sensations without judgment. Notice the feeling of your body against the surface you're lying on, the warmth or coolness, any areas of tightness, or any areas that feel relaxed.

6. **Release Tension**: If you notice any areas of tension, see if you can consciously release that tension as you exhale. Imagine the tension melting away with each breath.

7. **Stay Present**: If your mind starts to wander, gently guide your attention back to the body scan. Allow yourself to fully immerse in the experience of observing your body.

8. **Complete the Scan**: Continue the body scan, moving down through your neck, shoulders, arms, chest, abdomen, hips, legs, and finally down to your toes.

9. **Full Body Awareness**: Once you've completed the body scan, take a moment to bring your awareness to your body as a whole. Feel the sensations throughout your entire body.

10. **Ending the Practice**: When you're ready to end the practice, take a few deep breaths. Gently wiggle your fingers and toes, gradually bringing awareness back to your surroundings. Open your eyes if they were closed.

Mindful Walking

This exercise involves taking a mindful walk, which can be a wonderful way to connect with your surroundings and stay present. Find a safe and quiet place to walk, either indoors or outdoors, and let's begin:

1. **Begin Walking**: Start walking at a comfortable pace. It doesn't matter if it's a short distance; what matters is your intention to be fully present during the walk.

2. **Focus on Your Steps**: As you walk, bring your attention to the sensation of your steps. Notice the contact your feet make with the ground. Feel the shifting of your weight from one foot to the other.

3. **Observe Your Body**: Pay attention to how your body moves as you walk. Feel the rhythm of your arms swinging by your sides. Notice your posture and how your body responds to each step.

4. **Engage Your Senses**: Use your senses to fully experience the walk. Notice the temperature of the air, any breeze against your skin, and the sounds around you. Be present with the sights, sounds, and sensations of the environment.

5. **Notice Your Thoughts**: As you walk, thoughts may arise. Instead of getting caught up in these thoughts, view them as passing clouds. Gently redirect your attention back to the physical experience of walking and your surroundings.

6. **Breathe Mindfully**: As you walk, synchronize your breath with your steps. Inhale for a few steps, and then exhale for a few steps. This helps anchor your attention to your breath and the present moment.

7. **Stay Open and Curious**: Approach your walk with a sense of curiosity. Notice details you might not have noticed before. Explore the texture of the ground, the colors of nature, or the architecture around you.

8. **Full Presence**: Be fully present with each step. Allow the walk to become a moving meditation, where your focus is on the experience of walking itself.

9. **Complete Your Walk**: When you're ready to end the walk, gradually slow down your pace. Take a few moments to stand still and simply observe your surroundings.

10. **Reflect and Transition**: Take a moment to reflect on how you feel after the mindful walk. Notice any changes in your state of mind or body. Carry this sense of presence and calm with you as you transition back to your daily activities.

Gratitude Journaling

This activity, which consists of writing in a notebook and thinking on the things for which you are thankful might assist you in shifting your attention to the more positive elements of your life. Find a quiet and comfortable place to sit with a notebook or journal, and let's get started:

1. **Prepare Your Journal**: Open your journal to a blank page. Have a pen or pencil ready.

2. **Set the Intention**: Take a moment to set the intention for this practice. Decide how many things you want to list that you're grateful for, whether it's three, five, or more.

3. **Breathe and Center**: Close your eyes and take a few deep breaths to center yourself. Allow any tension to release with each exhale.

4. **Start Gratitude Journaling**: Begin writing down the things you're grateful for. These can be big or small, simple or complex. Focus on the present moment as you list your items.

5. **Engage Your Senses**: As you write, engage your senses. Reflect on the sensations, emotions, and experiences associated with each thing you're grateful for.

6. **Stay Present**: As you write, let go of any distractions and immerse yourself in the process. Allow each item to evoke a sense of appreciation.

7. **Reflect on Details**: For each item on your list, take a moment to reflect on specific details. Why are you grateful for it? How does it enrich your life?

8. **Express Sincerity**: As you write, express genuine gratitude. Feel the emotion behind your words and allow yourself to connect deeply with the things you're listing.

9. **Explore Diverse Aspects**: Aim to include a diverse range of things in your list. This could include relationships, experiences, personal qualities, or even moments from your day.

10. **Reflect on Your List**: After you've completed your list, take a moment to read it over. Allow the feelings of gratitude and positivity to wash over you.

11. **Closure**: When you're ready, gently close your journal. Carry the sense of gratitude and presence you've cultivated with you as you continue your day.

Self-Compassion Break

This exercise combines mindfulness and self-compassion to help you respond to challenging moments with kindness and understanding. Find a quiet and comfortable place to sit, and let's begin:

1. **Pause and Breathe**: Take a moment to pause whatever you're doing. Close your eyes if you're comfortable, and take a few deep, calming breaths. Allow yourself to relax.

2. **Acknowledge Your Experience**: Bring to mind a situation or challenge that's been causing you stress, discomfort, or frustration. Acknowledge what you're feeling without judgment. This is a moment of self-awareness.

3. **Offer Yourself Kindness**: As you breathe, silently offer yourself kind and compassionate words. You might say to yourself, "May I be kind to myself. May I be patient. May I give myself the compassion I need."

4. **Feel the Words**: As you repeat these phrases, let the intention behind them resonate with you. Feel the warmth and gentleness of your own words as if you were offering comfort to a dear friend.

5. **Connect with Common Humanity**: Recognize that challenges and difficulties are a part of the human experience. You're not alone in facing these struggles. Silently tell yourself, "Others have felt this way too."

6. **Broaden Your Perspective**: Expand your awareness to consider that countless others have faced similar challenges. You're connected to a larger community of humanity that understands suffering and seeking comfort.

7. **Extend Kindness to Others**: As you breathe, imagine sending the same kind and compassionate phrases to someone you care about—a friend, family member, or loved one. Picture them receiving these words of kindness.

8. **Feel the Connection**: Sense the shared humanity between you and others. Recognize that everyone, including yourself, experiences difficulties and deserves compassion.

9. **Return to Yourself**: Bring your attention back to your own experience. Breathe in the sense of connection and compassion you've cultivated.

10. **Open Your Eyes**: When you're ready, open your eyes if they were closed. Take a moment to reflect on how this practice has affected your perspective and your present moment.

Mindful Eating
This exercise encourages you to bring your full attention to the act of eating, allowing you to savor your food and engage with your senses. Choose a snack or a small meal, and find a quiet space to sit down and eat without distractions:

1. **Choose Your Food**: Select a piece of food or a small portion of a meal to eat mindfully. It could be a piece of fruit, a handful of nuts, or any snack you enjoy.

2. **Set the Scene**: Find a comfortable place to sit down. Turn off any distractions such as the TV, phone, or computer. Create a peaceful environment for your mindful eating experience.

3. **Engage Your Senses**: Before you start eating, take a moment to observe the food with your eyes. Notice its color, shape, and texture. Engage your sense of sight fully.

4. **Feel the Texture**: Pick up the food and feel its texture between your fingers. Notice any sensations, temperature, or moisture.

5. **Smell the Aroma**: Bring the food close to your nose and take a deep breath to inhale its aroma. Allow the scent to fill your senses.

6. **Taste with Awareness**: Slowly take a small bite of the food. Focus on the taste, texture, and flavors. Chew slowly and deliberately, noticing how the taste evolves with each bite.

7. **Observe Your Chewing**: Pay attention to the process of chewing. Feel the movement of your jaw, the way the food breaks down, and how your tongue interacts with the flavors.

8. **Savor the Experience**: As you continue eating, savor each bite mindfully. Engage with the sensations and flavors as fully as possible.

9. **Notice Your Thoughts**: As you eat, thoughts might arise about the food, other things, or even judgments about the experience. Simply observe these thoughts without judgment and gently return your focus to the act of eating.

10. **Eat Slowly**: Take your time to eat the entire portion mindfully. Be fully present with each bite, and let the experience of eating unfold naturally.

11. **Reflect on the Experience**: When you finish eating, take a moment to reflect on how the mindful eating experience was different from your usual eating habits. Notice any changes in your awareness or connection with the food.

Body-Focused Meditation

This exercise helps you tune into the sensations of your body, fostering a strong connection to the present moment. Locate a spot that's free from disturbances where you are able to sit or lay down, and let's begin:

1. **Settle In**: Take a seat or lie down in a position that is suitable for you. To help you unwind, try shutting your eyes for a couple of minutes and taking some slow, deep breaths.

2. **Body Scan**: Start by bringing your attention to your toes. As you focus on each body part, notice any sensations—warmth, coolness, tingling, or even the absence of sensation. Slowly

move your attention up through your feet, ankles, calves, knees, and so on, until you reach the top of your head.

3. **Stay Present**: As you scan through each body part, avoid analyzing or judging the sensations. Simply observe and acknowledge what you feel.

4. **Areas of Tension**: When you encounter areas of tension or discomfort, spend a little extra time there. Breathe into these areas and imagine the tension melting away with each exhale.

5. **Breath Awareness**: After completing the full body scan, bring your focus to your breath. Observe the inherent rhythm of your breath as you breathe in and breathe out. Feel the rise and fall of your chest or the sensation at your nostrils.

6. **Body Awareness and Breath**: Combine your awareness of your body with your breath. As you inhale, imagine your breath flowing to any areas of tension or discomfort, soothing and relaxing them. As you exhale, imagine releasing any stress or discomfort with your breath.

7. **Mindful Observance**: If your mind starts to wander, gently guide your focus back to the sensations in your body and the rhythm of your breath.

8. **Non-Judgmental Awareness**: Throughout the practice, maintain a non-judgmental attitude toward the sensations you experience. Be open and curious about what you observe.

9. **Closing the Practice**: When you're ready to conclude, take a few deep breaths and gradually bring your awareness back to the room. Gently open your eyes if they were closed.

Chapter 5

The Journey Towards Lasting Well-being

Cumulative Benefits: How Consistency Leads to Reduced Stress and Enhanced Mood

Consistency plays a crucial role in reducing stress and enhancing mood through vagus exercises. By engaging in activities that stimulate the vagus nerve, you can activate the body's relaxation response, leading to reduced stress and improved mood.

Vagus exercises, like deep breathing, meditation, yoga, and progressive muscle relaxation, help to activate the vagus nerve and promote a state of calmness and relaxation. Here's how consistency in practicing these exercises can lead to reduced stress and enhanced mood:

1. **Neuroplasticity**: Consistently engaging in vagus exercises can lead to neuroplastic changes in the brain. Neuroplasticity is the capacity of the brain to restructure itself and change its function through the formation of new neural connections. Regular practice of vagus exercises can strengthen the connections associated with relaxation and emotional regulation, making it easier for the brain to respond to stress in a more balanced and composed manner.

2. **Habit Formation**: Consistency leads to habit formation. When you make vagus exercises a regular part of your routine, they become ingrained habits. This means that your body and mind become accustomed to the relaxation response triggered by these exercises. Over time, your body will be more inclined to respond to stressors with a calmer demeanor, leading to reduced stress levels overall.

3. **Stress Hormone Regulation**: Engaging in vagus exercises on a consistent basis helps regulate stress hormones like cortisol. These exercises promote the activation of the parasympathetic nervous system, which counteracts the "fight or flight" response associated with stress. By consistently activating the relaxation response, your body becomes better equipped to manage and balance stress hormone levels.

4. **Emotional Regulation**: The vagus nerve is connected to brain regions responsible for emotional regulation and mood control. Regular vagus exercises can lead to improved emotional regulation and enhanced mood stability. As you become more adept at shifting from a stressed state to a relaxed state, your overall emotional well-being improves.

5. **Reduced Inflammation**: Chronic stress is associated with increased inflammation in the body, which can undesirably impact both physical and mental health. Consistent vagus exercises have been shown to reduce inflammation by activating the cholinergic anti-inflammatory pathway, which is regulated by the vagus nerve. By mitigating inflammation, these exercises contribute to a healthier body and mind.

Consistency in practicing vagus exercises helps build a foundation of relaxation and resilience. By repeatedly stimulating the vagus nerve and activating the body's relaxation response, you create positive physiological and psychological changes that lead to reduced stress and enhanced mood. It's important to note that while consistency is key, individual experiences may vary, and it's advisable to consult with a healthcare professional before making important changes to your routine, especially if you have underlying health conditions.

Setting Goals and Tracking Progress: Your Path to Well-being

Setting goals and tracking progress are like your companions on the road to a happier, healthier you, especially when it comes to doing vagus nerve exercises. Think of goals as the destinations you want to reach on this journey. They're like signposts that guide you and keep you focused. These destinations can be simple, like feeling less stressed, or specific, like boosting your mood. Making your goals clear and achievable is important. For instance, if you're new to vagus nerve exercises, a goal could be doing a quick deep-breathing exercise for a few minutes each day.

Goals give you a purpose, a reason to keep moving forward. When you have a goal in mind, it's like having a mission that motivates you. It's easier to stay committed and overcome obstacles when you know what you're working towards. Vagus nerve exercises have this wonderful power to relax you, reduce stress, and make you feel better overall. When you set goals for these exercises, it's like pointing a spotlight on their benefits, making them even more effective.

Now, imagine your well-being journey as a path you're traveling on. Tracking progress is like looking back at the path you've walked and seeing how far you've come. It's a way to see the progress you've made and to make sure you're on the right track. To track progress, you can keep a simple record. It could be a diary where you jot down when you did your vagus exercises, or a calendar where you put a mark on the days you completed your routine.

Tracking progress is like watching a story unfold. It's a visual reminder of all the days you've worked on your goals. When you see the marks add up or the pages fill with your efforts, it's a boost of motivation. It's like a little pat on the back, telling you that you're doing great. Tracking your vagus exercises lets you see how they slowly make a difference in your stress levels and mood. It's like watching the puzzle pieces of your well-being come together.

Here's how it all connects: setting goals gives you a direction, a purpose for your vagus exercises. It's like having a map that guides you on this journey. And tracking progress is like having a compass that shows you the direction you're heading in. Your vagus exercises are like tools in your backpack, helping you get closer to your goals. By doing these exercises regularly, you're actually telling your body to relax. This can lower stress and make you feel happier. And when you track your practice, you can see how these little exercises add up to something big for your well-being.

Now, let's get practical. Starting small is key. Begin with goals that you know you can reach. Maybe it's just a few minutes of vagus exercises each day. Setting a routine helps too. Pick a time, like in the morning or before bed, and stick to it. Reminders can be a great help until the exercises become a habit. You can set an alarm or put a note where you'll see it. Celebrate the small wins. When you see your progress adding up, take a moment to pat yourself on the back. And be patient. Results take time. So, don't rush. Trust that your efforts will show results.

Setting goals and tracking progress are like your guides on the journey to well-being, especially when it comes to doing vagus nerve exercises. Goals give you a direction and a purpose, making your exercises more effective. Tracking progress is like watching your efforts turn into something amazing. By making these practices a part of your daily life, you're taking steps towards a better you. And remember, small steps today lead to big changes tomorrow.

Write below your goals for the next year

- January

- February

- March

- April

- May

- June

- July

- August

- September

- October

- November

- December

____

____

____

Chapter 6

Tailoring Your Approach

Diverse Techniques for Diverse Preferences: Breathing, Movement, and Grounding

People have diverse preferences when it comes to maintaining their well-being, and fortunately, there are various techniques that cater to these differences. Three widely used methods are breathing exercises, movement practices, and grounding techniques. These approaches offer unique benefits and can be tailored to individual preferences and needs.

Breathing Exercises: Breathing is a vital aspect of human life, and certain breathing techniques can profoundly impact mental and emotional states. Deep breathing, also known as diaphragmatic breathing, involves taking slow, deliberate breaths that engage the diaphragm. This technique activates the parasympathetic nervous system, promoting relaxation and reducing stress. Alternate nostril breathing, a yogic practice, helps balance energy and enhance focus. Box breathing involves inhaling, holding, exhaling, and holding again for equal counts, which can help stabilize emotions. Breath awareness meditation encourages mindful observation of the breath, promoting a calm and centered state of mind. Breathing exercises are versatile and can be practiced anywhere, making them an accessible option for managing stress and anxiety.

Movement Practices: Movement-based techniques offer a dynamic approach to well-being. Yoga combines physical postures, breath control, and meditation to improve flexibility, strength, and mental clarity. Tai Chi, an ancient Chinese practice, emphasizes slow, flowing movements that enhance balance, coordination, and relaxation. Dance therapy combines movement and emotional expression, providing an outlet for creativity and self-discovery. Cardiovascular exercises like running or cycling release endorphins, improving mood and reducing stress. These movement practices cater to those who find solace and rejuvenation through physical activity, providing an avenue for self-care that aligns with their preferences.

Grounding Techniques: Grounding techniques connect individuals with the present moment and their surroundings, helping alleviate anxiety and stress. Mindful awareness involves focusing on the senses—sight, sound, touch, smell, and taste—to anchor oneself in the current experience. Progressive muscle relaxation entails tensing and then releasing different muscle groups, promoting physical relaxation. Visualization techniques guide individuals through imagined scenarios, fostering relaxation and positivity. Nature-based grounding encourages spending time outdoors, connecting with the natural world to restore balance. These techniques resonate with those who seek a sense of stability and presence in their self-care routines.

Incorporating these techniques into your self-care regimen can have a transformative impact on your well-being. However, it's important to recognize that personal preferences vary, and what works for one person may not work for another. Experiment with different techniques to discover which resonate with you the most. Furthermore, consider combining these approaches for a comprehensive self-care routine that addresses different aspects of your physical, mental, and emotional health.

Ultimately, the key to effective self-care is understanding your needs, being open to exploration, and customizing your approach to match your preferences. By embracing a diverse range of techniques—whether it's through breathing exercises, movement practices, grounding techniques, or a combination of these—you can create a holistic self-care routine that supports your well-being in a way that feels personally fulfilling and sustainable.

Communication and Connection: Sharing Your Self-Care Needs

When it comes to taking care of yourself amidst the hustle and bustle of life, sharing your self-care needs with others is a vital step in ensuring your mental, emotional, and physical well-being. To effectively communicate your needs, begin by reflecting on what those needs truly entail. Think about the aspects of your life that require attention and the activities that help you recharge and find balance. Once you've identified your needs, choose the right time and place to have this conversation. Find a quiet and comfortable space where you can talk openly without distractions, and make sure both you and the person you're communicating with are in a receptive state.

Honesty and directness are key components of effective communication. Express your self-care needs openly and honestly, explaining why they are important to you. Share how neglecting self-care can impact your overall well-being, using "I" statements to express your feelings and needs without coming across as confrontational. As you express your needs, remember to also set boundaries. Let others know about behaviors or situations that drain you, and propose alternatives. If you need alone time to recharge, emphasize that it's about your personal well-being rather than a reflection on your relationship with them.

Listening actively is just as important as expressing your needs. After conveying your thoughts, attentively listen to the other person's response. They might have questions or concerns that deserve your consideration. Engage in a genuine dialogue to foster mutual understanding. While it's important to prioritize your self-care needs, being open to compromise is essential in maintaining healthy relationships. Find middle ground that suits both parties, taking into account everyone's needs.

Consider using this opportunity to educate others about the significance of self-care and its benefits. Not everyone may fully grasp the concept, so sharing insights can help them better understand and support your efforts. When discussing your self-care needs, it's crucial to manage expectations. Clarify that self-care isn't about shirking responsibilities, but rather about ensuring you're in the best position to fulfill them. Strike a balance between advocating for your well-being and maintaining a respectful tone.

Lastly, show appreciation for the support and understanding you receive after discussing your self-care needs. Acknowledge the effort others put into accommodating your needs and assure them that your well-being enhances your relationships. Remember that sharing your self-care needs is an ongoing process. People may not fully comprehend your needs right away, but consistent communication can lead to positive changes over time. By openly expressing your self-care needs, you prioritize your own well-being and pave the way for healthier, more fulfilling relationships with those around you.

Chapter 7

Embracing a Holistic Lifestyle

The Connection: Vagus Nerve Health and Holistic Well-being

The human body operates as a complex mechanism with a range of processes and systems, among which the vagus nerve plays a pivotal role. Although often overlooked, the vagus nerve is a vital element within the human body. Its responsibilities encompass the regulation of critical bodily functions such as heart rate, breathing, and digestion. Additionally, it exerts a profound influence on mental health and overall well-being.

Dr. Nicole LePera, a Holistic Psychologist, emphasizes that the vagus nerve serves as the cornerstone of the entire nervous system. Acting as the overseer of the parasympathetic nervous system, it manages the rest and digestion processes that are essential for both mental and physical well-being. Dr. LePera often refers to the vagus nerve as the "wandering nerve" due to its extensive reach throughout the body. This nerve serves as a connecting link between the brain and vital organs like the digestive system, lungs, heart, liver, and spleen.

When the vagus nerve operates optimally, its impact on mental health is profound. Conversely, dysfunction in the vagus nerve can contribute to various mental health challenges, comprising anxiety, depression, and even post-traumatic stress disorder (PTSD).

Dr. Glenn Doyle, a clinical psychologist, elucidates that the vagus nerve is frequently referred to as the "brain-gut" axis due to the strong connection between the gut and the brain. This connection explains the sensation of "butterflies" in the stomach during periods of nervousness or anxiety. Stimulation of the vagus nerve offers the potential to alleviate anxiety and depression by calming the nervous system and fostering relaxation.

While the vagus nerve might not be a familiar term for many, its undeniable impact on both physical and mental well-being underscores its significance. This nerve plays a foundational role in regulating diverse bodily functions, encompassing digestion, heart rate, and cognitive processes. Neglecting the health of the vagus nerve can lead to adverse outcomes, including heightened stress, anxiety, and other mental health challenges. Yet, by incorporating daily practices that stimulate the vagus nerve, such as deep breathing, meditation, and yoga, individuals can cultivate relaxation, alleviate anxiety and depression, and advance overall mental and physical health. By attending to the vagus nerve, individuals can assume control over their physical and mental well-being, fostering a more gratifying and fulfilling life.

Nurturing Your Body, Mind, and Spirit

Nurturing your body, mind, and spirit through vagus nerve exercises can have a positive impact on your overall well-being. By engaging in activities that stimulate and activate the vagus nerve, you can promote relaxation, reduce stress, and enhance your overall health. Here's a guide on how to nurture these aspects of yourself through vagus nerve exercises:

1. **Deep Breathing:** Practice deep, diaphragmatic breathing. Take slow and deep breaths, filling your abdomen as you breathe in and letting it contract as you breathe out. This breathing technique activates the vagus nerve and can help alleviate stress and anxiety.

2. **Meditation and Mindfulness:** Engage in regular meditation or mindfulness practices. These practices can help calm the mind, reduce stress, and promote a sense of well-being. Focus on your breath, bodily sensations, or a specific mantra to activate the vagus nerve.

3. **Cold Exposure:** Taking cold showers or immersing yourself in cold water can stimulate the vagus nerve. The shock of cold exposure triggers a response known as the "diving reflex," which helps regulate heart rate and promotes relaxation.

4. **Singing or Chanting:** Engage in activities that involve singing, humming, or chanting. The vibrations produced by these activities can stimulate the vagus nerve and improve mood.

5. **Laughter:** Laughter is known to have a positive impact on the vagus nerve. Partake in activities that bring out laughter, like watching a comedic movie or hanging out with friends who bring happiness to your world.

6. **Yoga:** Certain yoga poses and practices, such as the "cobra" or "fish" poses, involve backbending and opening the chest, which can stimulate the vagus nerve. Yoga also promotes relaxation and reduces stress.

7. **Breathing Exercises:** Engage in specific breathing exercises designed to stimulate the vagus nerve. One example is the "4-7-8" breathing technique, where you inhale for a count of 4, hold for a count of 7, and exhale for a count of 8.

8. **Social Connection:** Engage in meaningful social interactions with friends, family, and loved ones. Positive social interactions have been shown to activate the vagus nerve and improve emotional well-being.

9. **Positive Emotions:** Cultivate positive emotions such as gratitude, compassion, and joy. These emotions have been linked to increased vagal tone, which reflects the health and responsiveness of the vagus nerve.

10. **Aerobic Exercise:** Regular aerobic exercises, such as swimming, jogging, or cycling, can increase vagal tone and overall parasympathetic nervous system activity.

Remember that consistency is key when practicing vagus nerve exercises. Include these activities into your daily routine and give yourself time to experience their benefits.

Chapter 8:

Enhancing Your Knowledge

Safeguarding Your Journey: Essential Safety Precautions

Engaging in vagus nerve exercises can offer numerous benefits for overall well-being, but it's important to approach these practices with caution to ensure safety and effectiveness. To make the most of these exercises while safeguarding your health, it's essential to adhere to a set of safety precautions.

1. **Consultation with a Healthcare Professional:** Before embarking on any new exercise regimen, especially those that involve physiological changes like vagus nerve stimulation, it's crucial to consult a healthcare professional. This is particularly important if you have any pre-existing medical conditions, such as cardiovascular issues, respiratory problems, or neurological disorders.

2. **Gradual Progression:** Start slowly and gradually increase the intensity and duration of your vagus nerve exercises. Rapid or excessive stimulation could potentially lead to adverse reactions, such as dizziness or fainting. Gradual progression lets your body adapt and minimizes the risk of discomfort.

3. **Listen to Your Body:** Pay close attention to how your body responds during and after vagus nerve exercises. If you encounter any uncommon symptoms like chest pain, difficulty breathing, feeling dizzy, or nausea, halt the exercises right away and, if necessary, seek medical assistance.

4. **Breathing Techniques:** When practicing deep breathing exercises, ensure that you're not hyperventilating. Overbreathing can disrupt the balance of oxygen and carbon dioxide in your blood, leading to adverse effects. Aim for slow, controlled breaths to maintain proper physiological balance.

5. **Comfortable Posture:** Maintain a comfortable and safe posture during exercises like meditation and yoga. Avoid extreme positions that could strain your muscles or joints. If you have mobility concerns, consider modified poses or chairs for support.

6. **Avoid Overexertion:** While vagus nerve exercises can provide relaxation, pushing yourself too hard can have counterproductive effects. Striking a balance between gentle stimulation and overexertion is crucial for reaping the benefits without causing undue stress to your body.

7. **Hydration and Nutrition:** Stay adequately hydrated before and after your exercises. Proper hydration supports overall bodily functions and helps prevent complications. Additionally, having a light meal or snack before exercises can help stabilize blood sugar levels and provide the energy needed for the session.

8. **Mindfulness and Emotional Awareness:** Vagus nerve exercises often involve relaxation and emotional regulation. Be mindful of any emotions that arise during these exercises. If you experience intense emotional reactions, it's important to approach them with self-compassion and seek professional support if necessary.

9. **Individual Differences:** Remember that everyone's response to vagus nerve exercises can vary based on factors such as age, health status, and genetics. What works well for one person might not work the same way for another.

10. **Consistency and Long-Term Approach:** Consistency is valuable, but avoid becoming overly zealous. Instead of aiming for a high number of repetitions right away, focus on creating a sustainable, long-term routine that aligns with your body's capacity and needs.

Incorporating these safety precautions into your vagus nerve exercise routine will help you reap the rewards of enhanced relaxation, stress reduction, and emotional balance while minimizing the risk of potential adverse effects. Remember that your well-being is a priority, and taking the time to approach these exercises mindfully and responsibly will contribute to a positive and holistic experience.

Staying Grounded: Navigating Through Misconceptions

The vagus nerve has become a key focus in the journey toward overall well-being. The burgeoning interest in vagus nerve exercises as a means to alleviate stress, enhance mood, and improve overall health has led to a proliferation of information. Yet, amidst this wealth of knowledge, misconceptions often lurk, potentially hindering the efficacy of these exercises. Navigating through these misconceptions is essential to harness the true potential of vagus nerve exercises for well-being.

Misconception 1: One-Size-Fits-All Approach

A common fallacy is that a singular vagus nerve exercise can universally address well-being. In reality, individuals have varying physiological and psychological responses. What works for one person might not be equally effective for another. It is imperative to recognize the diversity of exercises available—ranging from deep breathing and meditation to yoga and cold exposure. Tailoring these exercises to one's own preferences and needs is crucial for optimizing results.

Misconception 2: Instant Gratification

In an era of rapid results, some believe that vagus nerve exercises yield immediate benefits. While these exercises can induce relaxation, their impact is often cumulative. Consistent practice over time is necessary to trigger lasting physiological changes that lead to reduced stress and improved mood. Patience is key; expecting instant transformation can lead to disillusionment and premature abandonment of the practice.

Misconception 3: Quantity Over Quality

Engaging in numerous vagus nerve exercises without paying heed to technique and intention can be counterproductive. Quality trumps quantity. Mindful engagement with each exercise ensures a deeper connection with the body and mind, facilitating the desired physiological response. Rushing through exercises in a checklist manner dilutes their efficacy and misses the essence of the practice.

Misconception 4: Disregarding Lifestyle Factors

A misconception often overlooked is that vagus nerve exercises exist in isolation from other lifestyle factors. Diet, sleep patterns, physical activity, and social connections profoundly influence vagal tone—the activity level of the vagus nerve. Neglecting these factors can impede progress. Combining vagus nerve exercises with a holistic approach to well-being enhances their impact.

Misconception 5: Ignoring Individuality

The belief that vagus nerve exercises are universally beneficial regardless of an individual's health condition is misleading. Certain medical conditions can influence the suitability of specific exercises. Consulting a healthcare professional before embarking on a regimen is crucial, especially for individuals with preexisting health concerns.

Misconception 6: Short-Term Commitment

Effective vagus nerve exercises demand consistency and long-term commitment. Viewing these exercises as a quick fix rather than an ongoing practice can hinder progress. Cultivating a routine that seamlessly integrates into daily life nurtures the mind-body connection over time.

Chapter 9:

The Power of Personal Stories

Real-life Anecdotes: How Vagus Nerve Exercises Transformed Lives

In the midst of our hectic lives, many individuals discover significant benefits from practicing daily vagus nerve exercises. These simple routines, designed to tap into a part of our nervous system linked to relaxation, have been making waves for their potential to bring a sense of calm to the storm of modern life. Let's dive into a few personal stories that show how these exercises have actually worked for real people, from reducing anxiety to getting better sleep and even facing social fears.

One remarkable story comes from Sarah, a 32-year-old marketing professional. Plagued by chronic anxiety for years, Sarah felt she had exhausted all conventional treatments. Intrigued by the growing buzz around vagus nerve stimulation, she decided to explore breathing exercises, which are known to activate the vagus nerve. Through consistent deep breathing and mindfulness practices, Sarah noticed her anxiety gradually receding. She recounted how, during a particularly stressful presentation, she employed these techniques and experienced a significant reduction in her usual anxiety symptoms, allowing her to deliver her talk confidently.

John, a 45-year-old executive, had battled with insomnia for decades. Sleep medications provided temporary relief but came with their own set of side effects. Frustrated, John delved into research on natural sleep aids and discovered the role of the vagus nerve in regulating sleep. He adopted a routine of daily yoga and meditation, practices that promote vagal tone—the responsiveness of the vagus nerve. Within weeks, John experienced a remarkable improvement in his sleep patterns. He marveled at how a few minutes of dedicated practice each day had transformed his nights, leaving him refreshed and energized.

The impact of vagus nerve exercises isn't limited to individual well-being; it extends to interpersonal relationships. Emily, a 28-year-old teacher, had always struggled with social anxiety. Simple interactions would trigger intense nervousness and panic. Learning about the vagus nerve's influence on social engagement, Emily embarked on a journey of self-improvement. She engaged in activities that required her to step out of her comfort zone, like attending social events and volunteering. Over time, her interactions became smoother, and she forged meaningful connections. Emily's story is a testament to how enhancing vagal tone can foster emotional resilience and nurture social bonds.

Digestive issues can also be alleviated through vagus nerve exercises, as evidenced by Michael's story. For years, Michael battled with irritable bowel syndrome (IBS), which hindered his daily life. Desperate for relief, he turned to vagus nerve exercises that promote gut-brain communication. Incorporating practices like diaphragmatic breathing and abdominal massages, Michael observed a significant reduction in his IBS symptoms. He could finally savor meals without fearing the ensuing discomfort. His experience underscores the profound link between vagal tone and digestive health.

These anecdotes collectively illuminate the life-transforming potential of vagus nerve exercises. From alleviating anxiety and insomnia to enhancing social interactions and digestive health, targeted practices hold the promise of reshaping lives. These personal stories also reflect the growing recognition of the mind-body connection in modern healthcare.

However, it's important to note that while these anecdotes are compelling, individual experiences can vary, and vagus nerve exercises might not yield the same results for everyone. Consultation with a healthcare professional is advisable before embarking on any new wellness regimen, particularly if one has pre-existing medical conditions. As research on the vagus nerve and its exercises continues to evolve, these anecdotes serve as inspirational narratives that highlight the potential for positive change through mind-body interventions.

Inspiring Change: Sharing Your Wellness Journey

Embarking on your wellness journey has been an inspiring experience filled with transformative moments. As you open up about your path to wellness, authenticity becomes your guiding light. Sharing your challenges and successes with honesty makes your journey relatable, reminding others that change is attainable even in the face of obstacles.

Start by delving into why you began this journey—what drove you to take those first steps? Let others glimpse the motivation that sparked your desire for better health, increased fitness, or mental well-being. By sharing your initial motivations, you help others connect with the roots of your transformation.

The milestones you've achieved along the way are not only personal victories but also sources of motivation for others. Detail your progress, from tangible achievements like reaching a fitness goal or adopting a healthier diet, to the subtle shifts like improved sleep quality and reduced stress levels. These moments of triumph show that progress is real and attainable.

Don't hesitate to dive into the strategies that have propelled your journey forward. Whether it's the routines you've established, the mindfulness techniques you've embraced, or the dietary changes you've made, your insights are valuable tools for others seeking to enact positive changes in their lives.

Let before-and-after visuals tell a visual story of your transformation. These photos can be compelling evidence of the progress you've made, encouraging those who are just starting out.

Your journey has undoubtedly had its share of obstacles. Sharing how you've navigated these challenges—be it conquering self-doubt, managing cravings, or juggling busy schedules—provides a roadmap for others encountering similar roadblocks.

The shifts in your mindset have been pivotal. Reflect on how you've cultivated a positive attitude, practiced self-kindness, and built resilience. These shifts often underpin the lasting changes in habits and lifestyle.

Engage with your audience, inviting them to share their stories and questions. By fostering a sense of community, you're creating a space where others can find support and inspiration.

Celebrate victories that aren't necessarily measured in numbers. Talk about the newfound self-confidence, enhanced self-esteem, and overall sense of well-being that have blossomed during your journey.

Your willingness to share your journey is an act of encouragement and support. Offer resources, recommend books, and provide guidance to those who may find your path inspiring. Remember, your journey has the potential to ignite change in others, creating a chain reaction of positive transformation that stretches far beyond your own experiences.

Chapter 10:

Evolving Through Feedback and Growth

Honoring Your Well-being: Addressing Feedback and Concerns

Engaging in vagus nerve exercises is a valuable strategy for promoting relaxation, reducing stress, and enhancing overall well-being. However, addressing feedback and concerns is essential to ensure that individuals can reap the full benefits of these exercises while minimizing potential challenges. With a growing interest in this practice, it's crucial to address common queries, provide guidance on overcoming obstacles, and highlight the importance of seeking professional advice when necessary.

1. **Understanding Vagus Nerve Exercises**

Vagus nerve exercises encompass a range of activities aimed at stimulating the vagus nerve, a crucial component of the parasympathetic nervous system. These exercises promote the relaxation response, leading to decreased heart rate, improved digestion, and reduced stress levels. Practices like deep breathing, meditation, yoga, and progressive muscle relaxation can effectively activate the vagus nerve.

2. **Common Concerns and Feedback**

As individuals venture into vagus nerve exercises, several common concerns and feedback may arise:

- **Frustration with Immediate Results:** Some individuals might anticipate instant outcomes from vagus nerve exercises, which can lead to frustration if rapid changes don't occur. It's important to emphasize that consistent practice over time yields the most substantial benefits.
- **Difficulty with Relaxation Techniques:** Certain relaxation techniques, like meditation, can be challenging for beginners who struggle with quieting their minds. Encouragement to start with shorter sessions and gradual progression can help overcome this challenge.

- **Physical Limitations:** Individuals with certain physical conditions may find specific exercises uncomfortable or unfeasible. Providing alternative exercises that are better suited to their abilities is essential.
- **Lifestyle Constraints:** Busy schedules and life commitments can impede consistent practice. Guiding individuals on integrating vagus exercises into their daily routines can help them overcome this hurdle.
- **Health Concerns:** People with pre-existing medical conditions or those on medication may have concerns about the potential effects of vagus exercises. Addressing these concerns underscores the importance of consulting healthcare professionals before starting any new regimen.

3. **Overcoming Challenges**

Addressing these concerns and feedback requires a comprehensive approach:

- **Education:** Educate individuals about the gradual nature of the benefits. Emphasize that just like physical exercise, consistent practice is key for long-term results.
- **Variety of Techniques:** Highlight the diversity of vagus nerve exercises available. Not all techniques work equally well for everyone, so individuals can explore and find what suits them best.
- **Mindfulness and Patience:** Encourage a mindful approach to the exercises. Acknowledge that progress might be gradual, and patience is crucial for achieving lasting changes.
- **Modification and Adaptation:** Offer modified exercises for those with physical limitations. Adapting poses or movements ensures that everyone can participate comfortably.
- **Integration into Routine:** Provide practical suggestions for integrating exercises into daily routines. This helps individuals carve out time for practice, making it more sustainable.
- **Professional Consultation:** Stress the importance of consulting healthcare professionals, particularly for individuals with medical conditions or those on medications. This ensures that any potential interactions or concerns are addressed effectively.

4. **Holistic Well-being**

Vagus nerve exercises are one facet of holistic well-being. Encourage individuals to complement these exercises with other healthy habits, such as balanced nutrition, regular exercise, and quality sleep, to optimize their overall well-being. Vagus nerve exercises offer a promising pathway to relaxation, stress reduction, and enhanced well-being. Addressing common concerns and feedback empowers individuals to embark on this journey with confidence. By providing guidance, education, and adaptability, practitioners can navigate potential obstacles and experience the transformative effects of these exercises. It's a reminder that every well-being journey is unique, and progress is achieved through consistency, patience, and informed decision-making.

Your Empowering Journey: Embracing a Lifelong Commitment

Embracing a lifelong commitment to practicing vagus nerve exercises can profoundly impact overall well-being. These simple yet powerful exercises can contribute to stress reduction, improved mood, and enhanced physical health. By consistently engaging in activities that activate the vagus nerve, you lay the foundation for a healthier and more balanced life.

Regular practice of vagus nerve exercises can gradually reduce stress levels. When stressors abound, the body's fight-or-flight response can be overwhelming. However, these exercises encourage the body to activate the parasympathetic nervous system, promoting relaxation and a sense of calm. Over time, this consistent activation helps the body respond more calmly to stressors.

Additionally, these exercises have the potential to uplift mood. By activating the vagus nerve, they stimulate the release of neurotransmitters like serotonin and dopamine, often referred to as "feel-good" chemicals. This can lead to improved emotional well-being, greater resilience, and a brighter outlook on life.

Consistency is key in reaping the benefits of these exercises. Much like tending to a garden, regular care nurtures growth. Just as watering plants daily leads to healthy blooms, engaging in vagus nerve exercises consistently nurtures a healthier mind and body. Developing a routine gradually ingrains these practices into your daily life, making them second nature.

Imagine the vagus nerve exercises as a toolbox for self-care. Much like you use tools to fix things around the house, these exercises serve as tools to mend and rejuvenate your well-being. By utilizing them consistently, you cultivate a toolkit for navigating life's challenges.

Moreover, these exercises need not be time-consuming or elaborate. Incorporating them into your routine can be as simple as taking a few minutes each day to breathe deeply, stretch, or meditate. The cumulative effect of these small actions can lead to profound changes over time.

In the grand journey of life, embracing a commitment to vagus nerve exercises is akin to choosing a healthier path. It's a choice to prioritize self-care and well-being. Just as a river shapes the land it flows through, these exercises shape your physical and emotional landscape, molding it into one of vitality and balance.

A lifelong commitment to vagus nerve exercises holds immense potential for transforming your well-being. With their stress-reducing, mood-enhancing, and health-promoting effects, these exercises are a simple yet invaluable tool. By consistently engaging in these practices, you invest in a healthier, more harmonious life—one where you can navigate challenges with resilience and embrace each day with a brighter spirit.

Conclusion: Empowering Your Inner Balance

In the journey to empower your inner balance, vagus nerve exercises stand as steadfast allies. These simple practices hold the key to unlocking a harmonious connection between your mind and body. By engaging in these exercises consistently, you create a bridge that spans the gap between the hustle and bustle of modern life and the calm sanctuary within you.

Think of vagus nerve exercises as a compass, guiding you back to your center amidst the chaos of daily life. They provide a respite, a chance to pause and recalibrate. As you breathe deeply, stretch gently, or meditate quietly, you're not just engaging in movements; you're embarking on a journey inward.

These exercises offer a tangible way to navigate stress's unpredictable tides. With each practice, you're activating the soothing power of the vagus nerve, a natural mechanism that gently eases your heart rate, steadies your breath, and invites tranquility. By consistently embracing these exercises, you're arming yourself with a shield against the storms of stress that may otherwise disrupt your equilibrium.

Furthermore, these exercises hold the key to amplifying your emotional harmony. They encourage the release of the body's own "feel-good" chemicals, fostering a brighter outlook and a sense of emotional resilience. As you engage in these practices, you're weaving threads of positivity into the tapestry of your emotional landscape, infusing it with colors of hope and serenity.

Consistency is the anchor that holds the vessel of inner balance steady. Just as the moon's consistent pull shapes the tides, your commitment to these exercises shapes the ebb and flow of your well-being. By making them a part of your routine, you're nurturing your inner equilibrium day by day, like a gardener tending to a precious garden of serenity.

In a world that often demands rapid responses and constant engagement, vagus nerve exercises provide a sanctuary of stillness. They remind you that amidst the whirlwind of life, you possess the power to ground yourself in the present moment. By dedicating yourself to these practices, you're declaring that your inner balance matters, that it's worth cultivating, and that you deserve the gift of well-being.

Vagus nerve exercises are more than just movements; they're gateways to your inner balance. Through consistent engagement, they offer a lifeline to serenity amidst the chaos, a source of emotional upliftment, and a touchstone to anchor your well-being. As you embark on this journey of empowerment, remember that with each practice, you're nurturing the garden of your inner harmony—one breath, one stretch, and one moment of stillness at a time.

Bonus

Unlock a world of mindfulness! Scan the QR code for an exclusive download of our eBook, a companion guide to 'Daily Vagus Nerve Exercises.' Immerse yourself in the essence of mindfulness, exploring techniques to cultivate presence, manage stress, and enhance your well-being. Your journey to a more mindful and balanced life begins with a simple scan. Embrace the transformative power of mindfulness today!

Your diary

Report here your progress and thoughs and keep track of your successes and difficulties. It will motivate you to keep going on and improve your life !